To Mum and Dad,

with love from the
editor!

Sarah

31.10.83

MODERN NURSING SERIES

General Editors

SUSAN E NORMAN, SRN, NDN Cert, RNT
Tutor for Staff Development, The Nightingale School, St Thomas'
Hospital, London

JEAN HEATH, BA, SRN, SCM, Cert Ed
National Health Learning Resources Unit,
Sheffield City Polytechnic

Consultant Editor

A J HARDING RAINS, MS, FRCS
Regional Dean, British Postgraduate Medical Federation, formerly
Professor of Surgery, Charing Cross Hospital Medical School, Honorary
Consultant to the Army

This series caters for the needs of a wide range of nursing, medical and
ancillary professions. Some of the titles are given below, but a complete list is
available from the Publisher.

Community Health and Social Services
J B MEREDITH DAVIES

Nursing—Image or Reality?
MARGARET C SCHURR and JANET TURNER

Communicable Diseases
WILFRID H PARRY

Gerontology and Geriatric Nursing
SIR W FERGUSON ANDERSON, F I CAIRD, R D KENNEDY and
DORIS SCHWARTZ

Obstetrics and Gynaecology
JOAN M E QUIXLEY and MICHAEL D CAMERON

Taverner's Physiology
DERYCK TAVERNER

Textbook of Surgery
R E HORTON

Intensive Care
A K YATES, P J MOORHEAD and A P ADAMS

COMMUNITY CHILD HEALTH

Marion E Jepson

MBE, MB, ChB, DCH, DPH, FFCM

Formerly Specialist in Community Medicine
(Child Health), Sheffield Health Authority

HODDER AND STOUGHTON
LONDON SYDNEY AUCKLAND TORONTO

The cover photograph was taken at the
Waterlea Adventure Playground, Crawley

British Library Cataloguing in Publication Data

Jepson, Marion E.
  Community child health.
  1. Community health services for children—
  Great Britain
  I. Title
  362.1'9892'000941   RJ103.G7

  ISBN 0 340 33285 9

First published 1983

Copyright © 1983 M. E. Jepson

All rights reserved. No part of this publication may be reproduced
or transmitted in any form or by any means, electronic, or mechanical,
including photocopy, recording, or any information storage or retrieval
system, without permission in writing from the publisher.

Typeset 10/11pt Times (Monophoto) by Macmillan India Ltd, Bangalore

Printed in Great Britain for Hodder and Stoughton Educational,
a division of Hodder and Stoughton Ltd,
Mill Road, Dunton Green, Sevenoaks, Kent TN13 2YD, by
Biddles Ltd, Guildford, Surrey

Editors' Foreword

This well established series of books reflects contemporary nursing and health care practice. It is used by a wide range of nursing, medical and ancillary professions and encompasses titles suitable for different levels of experience from those in training to those who have qualified.

Members of the nursing professions need to be highly informed and to keep critically abreast of demanding changes in attitudes and technology. The series therefore continues to grow with new titles being added to the list and existing titles being updated regularly. Its aim is to promote sound understanding by presenting essential facts clearly and concisely. We hope this will lead to nursing care of the highest standard.

Preface

Over the past century, children have been increasingly recognised as people in their own right with their own particular needs to be met. The great majority of children spend their life at home in the community, and this book attempts to set out some of the ways in which their health can be promoted and maintained.

Advances in preventive medicine, medical diagnosis and treatment have led to a decreasing incidence of many illnesses formerly known to be lethal or handicapping. There is now an accumulation of knowledge about the different aspects of development and the ways in which hereditary and environmental factors influence the well-being of the child and the extent to which he is able to achieve his potential. The tremendously important role of the parents is appreciated. Legislation to protect the child has proliferated and services of many kinds are available.

There still remains, however, a great concern that some children die, or are handicapped, or live in circumstances which diminish their prospects of well-being and happiness. The tasks involved in community child health work include a recognition that there are special individual health needs within the common needs of all children. The provision of services for child and family should be based on an evaluation of need and it is acknowledged that this can often best be met by a co-ordinated approach which 'enlists the parents as partners' and uses the contributions of many different agencies, both within the Health Service itself and other statutory and voluntary bodies.

The field of community child health is an immensely wide one and, within the limits of this book, it has not been possible to give full coverage to every aspect. Within the broad picture, some topics have been selected for more detailed consideration because they deal with commonly recurring situations which a professional health worker in the community meets, or because they illustrate some of the issues with which the community services are concerned.

The book is based on lectures given to students taking courses for the Certificate in Health Visiting, the Certificate of Social Work, the Midwifery Tutors Diploma, and to pupil midwives. It is hoped that it will be useful for nurses considering working in the community, and for those in hospital paediatric units whose concern for the child recognises the wider world in which he lives.

I am grateful to the following for permission to include illustrations: Miss K. Wall; Mr J. le Corney; the Sheffield Metropolitan District Environmental Health Department; Mr Colin New (Headmaster,

Hatfield House Lane FJM School, Sheffield); Mr C. C. Gold and Mr T. P. Highet (Headmasters of two special schools in Sheffield); the Sheffield Metropolitan District Education Department; Sheffield Health Authority and its Health Education Department; and the parents of the children whose photographs and writings are reproduced.

Many people have read individual chapters and I am most grateful for their helpful comments: Dr D. P. Adams, Miss M. Bourne, Miss J. Challinor, Professor J. Emery, Dr R. Mallet, Dr W. H. Parry, Dr R. M. Powell, Miss A. E. Salvin and Dr E. M. Taylor.

My thanks are due to Miss J. Dyson and Mrs. I. Ashton for the care and patience with which they have typed the text, and to Dr C. H. Shaw for his help with proof-reading.

Acknowledgements

The publisher wishes to acknowledge the following for giving permission to use their material in this book:

The Department of Health and Social Security for **Table 2.1** (from *Control of Communicable Diseases in Schools, DHSS/DES, 1977*) and **Table 2.3** (abstracted from *Immunisation against Infectious Disease, DHSS, 1982*); the Chief Medical Officer for **Fig. 2.1** (from the *Annual Reports of the CMO of the MoH/DHSS*); the Registrar General for **Figs. 3.1**, and **3.2**, and **Table 3.1** (based upon data from the *Registrar General's Annual Statistical Reviews of England and Wales* with the permission of the Controller of Her Majesty's Stationery Office; Crown copyright reserved); Her Majesty's Stationery Office for **Fig. 2.2** (from *Prevention of Health—Everybody's Business*) and **Fig. 3.3** (from *The House of Commons' Second Report of the Social Services Committee (Session 1979–80) Perinatal and Neonatal Mortality*); the Health Education Council for **Fig. 5.1** (from a leaflet published for Asian families) and **Fig. 8.4** (from a health education project to be published by Heinemann Educational Books in 1983); Sheffield Health Authority for **Table 2.4**.

Contents

Editors' Foreword		v
Preface		vi
Acknowledgements		vii
1	Child, Family and Environment	1
2	Prevention of Communicable Disease	18
3	Indices of Health	47
4	Surveillance of Health I — Growth in the Early Years	69
5	Surveillance of Health II — Other Aspects of Physical Health in the Early Years	85
6	Surveillance of Health III — Development in the Early Years	96
7	Surveillance of Health IV — School Children	109
8	Health Education	123
9	Services for Children	152
10	Children with Handicap	177
11	Children in Special Circumstances	206
12	Non-accidental Injury	222
13	Bereavement in the Family	232
14	The Future	237
Appendix—Recommended Reading		240
Index		244

1
Child, Family and Environment

The way in which a child grows and develops is the response to the interaction of two broad influences—the hereditary patterns initiated at the time of conception in the genes and chromosomes, and external influences acting throughout pregnancy and post-natal life which can be termed 'the environment'. A great deal has been written about the relative contribution of 'nature and nurture'. In the past, extremists have claimed the over-riding importance of either heredity or environment to the almost complete exclusion of the other, but today we are aware of many ways in which the two mechanisms interact and influence each other.

In attempting to assist a child to achieve his potential, it is necessary first of all to try to identify various factors, whether due to heredity or environment, which may influence his health, growth, and total development in physical, mental, social and emotional fields. Once identified, it may then be possible to encourage beneficial influences and avoid or counteract the harmful ones. Advances in knowledge of genetics have meant that heredity is no longer regarded as unalterable to the extent that it was in the past. Modern techniques of cytology and biochemical procedures, particularly those used in the examination of blood and amniotic fluid, have increased awareness of the effects of abnormal genes and chromosome formation; control of the spread of some undesirable hereditary factors is now possible through the detection of carriers and genetic counselling. Modern methods of therapy and management have improved the outlook in some inherited conditions (e.g. phenylketonuria and haemophilia). Nevertheless, the amount of change it is possible to effect, particularly once the child is born, is still relatively small. On the other hand, many environmental influences are capable (in theory at least) of alteration and amelioration. Their recognition is important, not only because of their direct effect on the health and well-being of children, but also because they may influence and modify the expression of hereditary factors—for example, a child's stature is the outcome of a genetically determined pattern and environmental factors such as family size and diet.

In recent years, concepts of what constitutes 'the environment' have broadened. The intra-uterine environment of the developing fetus now assumes considerable significance in relation to the importance of a good start in life. In post-natal life 'environment' is no longer confined to the relatively simple and easily defined influences such as housing, sanitation and food supply, but includes other elements found within the structure of the family itself (Fig. 1.1).

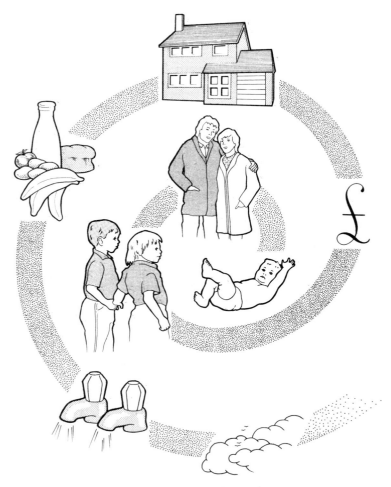

Fig. 1.1 The child and his environment

Pre-natal influences

These include the mother's health before and during pregnancy, the adequacy of her diet, freedom from infections such as rubella in early pregnancy, and personal habits (for example, smoking and alcohol intake), all of which can affect the intra-uterine environment in which the fetus develops. Modern ante-natal care, of which health education is an important component, recognises these influences and encourages parents-to-be to contribute in a positive way to giving their child a good start in life (Chapters 3 and 8).

Home

1 Parents

It is through the parents that the child first experiences his environment. Not only do they provide material care, but they also have the tremendous responsibility of meeting the basic needs of the growing child for love and affection, understanding and security. Poverty and poor housing may, and often do, add difficulties to the parents' task, but it is unwise to adopt material circumstances as the sole criterion of the quality of parental care. Love and security may abound in homes where the physical environment is far from satisfactory and, conversely, children brought up in homes of luxury may be deprived in other important ways. The expectations which parents have for their children's achievements vary a great deal. At one end of the scale, some parents expect very little and perhaps, through ignorance of a child's developmental needs for an environment of varied experience, toys, play, and language, do not provide sufficient stimulus. At the other extreme, too high and unrealistic expectations of behaviour and achievement may lead to stress in the child. Similarly the parents' norms of health and use of services vary according to their own experience, upbringing and the health standards of the community in which they live. Symptoms such as diarrhoea, upper respiratory tract infection and even convulsions, rightly regarded by many parents as reasons for seeking medical care, may be accepted by others as part of the usual pattern of childhood and of no untoward significance. Recent studies on infant deaths are showing that low norms of health may have a disastrous influence, not only on health but on life itself.

The last few years have seen a greater realisation of ways to help parents be good parents, to enjoy their children and understand their needs. Individual relationships with professional workers such as community nursing staff, social workers and advisory teachers, structured educational series arranged locally or through the media, and parent groups of many kinds all help to promote good child care.

2 Family size

Many children today are born into small families. This is a very different situation from 100 years ago, when a high infant death rate led to a large family often being regarded as a kind of insurance—a hope that at least some of the children would survive into adult life. The average family size today is 1–2 children per family. This reduction has come about for many reasons, which include the choice of the parents about family size, their expectations for their children's future, economic pressures, increased predicted survival of the children, awareness of rapid population growth, the availability of family planning services and the increased reliability of modern contraceptive methods. Small families may make possible many material benefits:

1   Couples can limit the size of their family in relation to the income available and so hope to provide a reasonable standard of living.
2   The effect of family size on growth as measured by height is striking: children in small families tend to be taller than those from large families.*
3   Housing problems are lessened.
4   There is the prospect of ensuring a longer period of full-time education for the children.
5   Parents are likely to be able to give more individual attention and stimulus and so encourage the child's mental and intellectual development.

On the other hand, it may be felt that the richness of experience of a different kind which comes from being a member of a large family could be missing in the small family. What is important is that couples should themselves be able to make considered decisions about their family size, in the light of their individual feelings and circumstances.

Family Planning   The NHS (Family Planning) Act of 1967 and subsequent associated acts emphasise the essential part that family planning can play in promoting family health and welfare and recognise the need to make services available to all, particularly in those instances where family limitation is an urgent social necessity. Through the National Health Service, family planning facilities are available free of charge from:

1   The general practitioner service.
2   Community family planning clinics.
3   The hospital services, which include family planning clinics associated usually with obstetric units, and provisions for vasectomy and female sterilisation.
4   Special centres which advise young people on personal problems of sex and contraception. These may be registered as charities, but are often subsidised by the National Health Service.
5   The domiciliary family planning service which many health authorities operate for those people who, for a variety of reasons, are unable or unwilling to come to a conventional clinic. This service is

---

*   from *Archives of Disease in Childhood*, **56**, no. 2, 1981

planned to take facilities into the home for women who have special difficulties in attending a clinic session.

A full range of contraceptives is available through the family planning services, and the choice of method for any client depends partly on individual preference, and partly on an assessment of the suitability of different methods in terms of reliability as a contraceptive measure, safety where general health is concerned, and acceptability to the woman and her partner. Modern contraceptive techniques such as long-acting hormonal preparations and intra-uterine devices, together with sterilisation, have facilitated successful family limitation, particularly where sustained individual responsibility is unreliable.

The fact that the number of births fell from 784 000 in 1970 to 569 800 in 1977 may be taken as a measure of family planning effectiveness, particularly as the decline was due mainly to a decrease of about a third in births to women of social classes IV and V (the partly skilled and unskilled workers). Nevertheless, in spite of the wide availability of free family planning services there is still evidence which points to numbers of unplanned and sometimes unwanted children being born. One of the major tasks of today and the future is to help couples make wise decisions about their family size, and to ensure that available services are known and fully used.

Family planning advice may be obtained from:

1 The general practitioner
2 Community clinics
3 Hospital clinics
4 Centres for young people
5 Domiciliary services

---

3 Family income

The association is well-established between an adequate family income with resulting ability to provide the many material necessities for children, and satisfactory standards of health and well-being. The provision of an adequate diet, clothing, warmth and reasonable housing conditions is dependent on a minimum amount of money coming into the home; an income on or below the poverty line may adversely influence many aspects of a child's life. The majority of children today grow up in families where material standards of living are adequate to meet basic needs. At any one time, however, there is a proportion of children growing up in single-parent families or families where poorly paid jobs, even with both parents working, barely provide a living wage; in other instances intermittent or permanent unemployment, redundancy and strikes may threaten standards of living. These circumstances are recognised in the continuous review of earnings in relation to the cost of living, and in the many schemes which have been introduced to relieve financial hardship in low income families.

Help for the low income family   Since 1948 there has been a series of measures designed to adjust some of the financial inequalities apparent in our society today. For parents, a number of benefits are available, some of which apply to all families regardless of income and others which are income-dependent.

Child benefit is a tax-free allowance, not means-tested, payable for each child, including the first, for whom a person is responsible. The benefit is available for all children under the age of 16 years (or under 19 if still at school or in a further educational establishment). An additional *one-parent benefit* may be claimed by a parent who has sole responsibility of bringing up a child or children.

Family income supplement (FIS) is intended for a family bringing up children on a low wage, and provides a means whereby the income of a family with at least one dependent child may be brought up to a level prescribed by Parliament. The availability of the supplement is limited to families where the man (or woman when she is the supporter of the family) is in full-time work. The amount granted depends on the family's gross income and the number of dependent children. Receipt of this supplement automatically entitles children to receive free school meals, and free milk and vitamins for those under school age.

Supplementary benefit is available for people not working full-time and who do not have enough to live on. The amount given depends on how much money the family is already getting and how much is needed weekly on which to live. Receipt of this benefit is also an entitlement to free school meals, free milk and vitamins and baby things.

Low income entitlements are available for people not receiving family income supplement or supplementary benefit but whose income fails to reach specific levels. The entitlements include free milk and vitamins for pre-school children.

Local Education Authorities may also grant free school meals and help in providing clothing and school uniform in cases of hardship.

Other benefits. The amount received from unemployment benefit, sickness benefit, widow's pension and invalidity pension varies with the number of dependent children.

Leaflets giving information on entitlement to benefits and how they may be claimed are available from social security offices.

> *Financial help for the family*
> 1 Child benefit
> 2 Family income supplement
> 3 Supplementary benefit
> 4 Low income entitlement
> 5 Help with school meals and clothing
> 6 Special allowances in other benefits

4 Housing

Housing plays a major part in the environment of children. Poor housing and overcrowding are associated particularly with:

1 An increased incidence of respiratory tract infections—colds, coughs, bronchitis and possibly asthma.
2 Increased risk of spread of communicable illness, particularly the common infections of childhood e.g. measles and whooping cough.
3 Increased risk of accidents e.g. scalds from kettles and burns from overturned paraffin heaters.
4 Mental stress in the parents—depression, tension and frustration which may precipitate non-accidental injury.
5 Cold hazards for the young baby.

Cold injury of the newborn   Very young babies, particularly if they are premature or of low birth-weight, are extremely susceptible to cold. Their physiological heat regulating mechanisms are not yet functioning adequately and if the body temperature falls too low (below 32°C/90°F), serious harm may result. The signs of a 'cold' baby develop gradually and include:

(a) Redness of the face which can be mistaken for a healthy colour.
(b) Redness and some hard oedema of the hands and feet.
(c) Coldness to the touch.
(d) Lethargy and difficulty in feeding.
(e) An unusually low temperature (special low-reading thermometers enable low body temperatures to be determined with accuracy).

Cold injury can be prevented by making sure that the temperature of the baby's room does not fall below 21°C/70°F day or night. Although cold rooms may be found in any home, particularly during the night, they are more likely in old houses with draughty doors and windows and inadequate heating facilities. The community midwife or health visitor will advise the mother about the provision of adequate clothing, cot coverings and additional heating. A baby who has become chilled should be warmed gradually and hospital admission is usually advised.

Because of the contribution to good health which satisfactory housing conditions make, improvement in housing has been one of the major concerns of the last few decades (Figs. 1.2 and 1.3). The local authority, through its environmental health and housing departments, has an important responsibility for ensuring that standards of housing are adequate.

Legal standards by which living conditions in houses and other dwellings are judged take into account:

1 *Structure*: the stability and state of repair of the house.
2 *Amenities* such as freedom from damp, adequate lighting, heating and ventilation, water supply, sanitary arrangements, facilities for the storage and cooking of food.
3 *Overcrowding*. These standards take into account the number of people of different ages and sex, living in one house and sharing basic facilities such as toilet and kitchen arrangements. They are particularly applicable to people living in rooms in houses in multiple occupation.

When houses are considered to be 'unfit for human habitation' the environmental health department has the authority to initiate measures which will either lead to the repair of the houses or restrict their use for

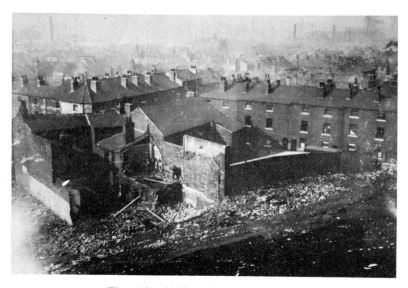

Fig. 1.2 Old housing—polluted air

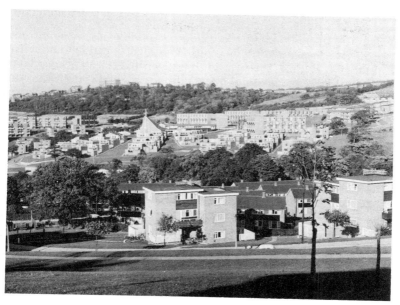

Fig. 1.3 New housing—clean air

accommodation. In the latter case, the housing department offers more suitable alternative housing for the occupants. New estates have been built to accommodate families and have provided a much higher standard of housing. Many are situated in pleasant surroundings at some distance from areas of heavy industry and provide all modern amenities in the way of indoor toilets and bathrooms, hot water, heating, cooking and storage facilities.

Undoubtedly modern material standards of housing have contributed a great deal to improved physical health, but some housing developments have not been without problems. Many young families rehoused in tower blocks or on estates on the outskirts of cities have experienced isolation from extended family and friends. Sometimes restriction of facilities for children, both indoors and outdoors, may deprive them of space for play—a valuable aid to development. High rents and fares to work may seriously deplete the family income. In the last few years, however, these drawbacks have been recognised and are now being taken into account in the planning stages of future housing developments.

Other housing policies, particularly in inner city areas, have placed the emphasis not necessarily on clearance of houses and rehousing at a distance but, wherever possible, on improving the standard of existing accommodation, thus enabling families to remain within a familiar neighbourhood with a well-established community spirit.

Help in housing

Rehousing. In addition to the rehousing of families living in unfit houses, most local authority housing departments operate some system of priority rehousing on medical grounds if it is felt that poor living conditions are contributing materially to a child's ill-health—for example, repeated severe respiratory infection thought to be aggravated by dampness, or a severely handicapped child living in a house without indoor toilet facilities.

Improvement grants. It is possible to obtain financial assistance for the improvement of certain houses, usually those lacking in the basic amenities of inside toilet, bathroom, hot water or adequate kitchen facilities. The grants, subject to certain conditions, are available for owner-occupiers and the owners of tenanted houses. Special grants are available for houses in multiple occupation.

Repair grants. Financial help is available at the discretion of the local council to enable repairs to be made to houses built before 1919.

Housing advice centres. These have been established in many areas and offer opportunities for discussion on individual housing problems, advice on mortgages and uptake of rent and rate rebates.

Rent and rate rebates. Direct financial help is available for tenants who cannot afford the full rent of their home. This includes families living in privately rented accommodation as well as those in council property, but does not include families already receiving supplementary benefit. The amount of the rebate varies according to the gross income of the family, the number of children and the rent payable. Similarly, rebates on the general rates, proportionate to income and family size, can be claimed from the local authority by owner-occupiers and tenants.

Both central Government and local authorities are very much aware of modern housing problems, and frequently review not only rehousing programmes but the extent to which different forms of financial help can be made available.

Help in housing

1 Rehousing
2 Improvement grants
3 Repair grants
4 Housing advice centres
5 Rent and rate rebates

The outside world

A number of environmental factors are controlled by measures which form part of the Government policy towards the promotion of healthy living. Many of these are concerned with safeguarding the health of total populations, but some have a special significance for children.

1   Food

Whilst the selection of food for a family is largely determined by availability, personal choice and the limitations of income, many legal measures protect the individual from buying food which could be unsafe or substandard.

Safety and Reliability of Food   Various legislative measures make it an offence for any food which is intended for human consumption to be offered for sale if it is likely to be injurious to health. The provisions not only cover perishable food but control, from a safety aspect, the many ways in which food today is processed to make it keep longer, appear attractive or simplify its use (e.g. preservatives, colouring matter, emulsifiers). The food hygiene regulations specify requirements regarding the cleanliness of premises of all kinds where food is stored, cooked or sold and stipulate standards of hygiene and health for people involved in the handling of food. These regulations are intended to reduce the risk of outbreaks of food poisoning amongst the general public. Many foods are required by law to conform to prescribed standards of composition in that their content and nutritional value, anticipated by the purchaser, is assured. The appropriate local authority is responsible for the enforcement of the measures.

Milk and its products form a valuable part of the diet of children and are subject to stringent safety regulations. In the past, infected milk has been responsible for tuberculosis, scarlet fever, haemolytic streptococcal throat infection, brucellosis, and salmonella infection. The problems of milk-borne disease have been greatly reduced by:

1   The establishment of herds free from tuberculosis and brucellosis.
2   The pasteurisation of milk.
3   Enforcement of adequate standards of hygiene in milking sheds, dairies and amongst milk-handlers.

The artificial feeding of small babies relies mainly on cows' milk which has been processed so as to make it, in many respects, comparable with human milk. Of particular importance is the amount of sodium (salt) in the feed reconstituted from dried milk. In the past, a combination of high sodium content in the powdered milk and difficulties in reconstituting the feed with a high level of accuracy resulted, at times, in too great a load being placed on the kidney. This is particularly dangerous in the very young baby because of consequent disturbance of the electrolyte balance of the blood (hypernatraemia). Modern manufacturing methods now enable dried milk with a safe sodium level to be produced and deaths in babies from hypernatraemia have been greatly reduced.

2   Water

99 % of the population in England and Wales receive piped water of a high degree of purity in their homes. The purification of water is a complex process involving storage and exposure to air, filtration and sterilisation to destroy organisms of intestinal origin, which might otherwise cause out-breaks of gastro-intestinal infections such as dysentery, typhoid and paratyphoid fevers. Responsibility for providing adequate and wholesome water supplies lies with the Water Authorities (collection, treatment and provision of supplies) and the local authorities (delivery of adequate pure water in pipes to houses and the purity of well- and spring-water for the 1 % of the population depending on this as their only source of water). Regular laboratory analysis of water is made, particular importance being placed on:

1   *Bacterial examination*, which establishes whether any excremental pollution has taken place. The number of bacteria of all kinds in a sample of water is counted, as well as any of faecal origin, and the findings are compared with standard indices of purity
2   *Chemical analysis*, which gives information regarding the hardness or softness of water and the concentration of certain minerals, particularly lead compounds and nitrates.

In this country, World Health Organisation (WHO) standards are used to determine the upper limit of safety for the chemical constituents of water.

Lead   Certain waters with an acid pH value, such as those originating in peaty moorlands, are capable of dissolving lead from lead piping and can contain a dangerously high lead level by the time the water reaches the consumer. A gradual replacement of old lead pipes with those of safer copper or plastic is diminishing this risk.

Nitrates   These are particularly important in relation to their effect, when in high concentrations, on babies in the first 12 weeks of life. Nitrates occur naturally in small amounts in most water supplies, but in some parts of the country the concentration may exceed the safety level; this is also likely to occur in any district in a period of drought. Under these circumstances young babies in the first months of life, taking artificial feeds made up with water, may take in appreciable amounts of nitrates which are later reduced to nitrites by the action of intestinal bacteria. The nitrites may then combine with the haemoglobin in the blood to form methaemoglobin.

Methaemoglobinaemia In this condition the oxygen-carrying capacity of the blood is reduced. Characteristic early signs are a slate-blue colour of the skin and cyanosis of the lips; clinical signs of a lack of oxygen may be seen at a later stage. Estimation of the methaemoglobin in a blood sample will confirm the diagnosis.

Treatment: The condition can be reversed by giving water of low nitrate content, but admission to hospital is usually recommended

Prevention: When water analysis shows high concentrations of nitrates, alternative supplies of low nitrate-content water should be made available to mothers with young bottle-fed infants. Mothers are also warned against prolonged boiling or re-boiling of water for feeds, which would increase the nitrate concentration.

Fluoride Much attention has been focused on the relationship between small amounts of fluoride in drinking water and the prevention of dental decay in children. Extensive research has shown that as little as one part fluoride per million parts drinking water is effective and in this concentration no harmful effects occur. Not all areas have naturally occurring fluoride in their water supply, and the Government is now encouraging the general introduction of fluoridation as an important preventive measure in dental health.

Swimming baths The purity of water in swimming baths is also carefully controlled as bacterial pollution could lead to intestinal, respiratory and ear infections. The standards for the bacterial content of water in baths are very strict.

Water is examined for:

1 Bacterial content
2 Chemical content: lead
                     nitrates
                     fluoride

---

3 Air

It is only in the past 25–30 years that the full importance of clean air in relation to health has been recognised. A number of studies have established the relationship between pollution and the incidence of lower respiratory tract infection in children, although there is still divided opinion as to the effect regarding upper respiratory tract infections. The Clean Air Act was introduced in 1956 and this restricted the amount of dark smoke permitted from factory emission and also made it possible for local authorities to enforce non-smoke-producing methods of heating for domestic purposes. These measures have produced major reductions in the amount of smoke and sulphur dioxide in the air, with a corresponding decrease in the incidence of lower respiratory tract infection in children, and have also contributed greatly to an improved aesthetic quality of the environment, particularly in the large industrial cities.

Lead merits special mention as an environmental hazard particularly relevant to children (Fig. 1.4). It has been mentioned briefly in connection with the lead content of water supplies, and there are also

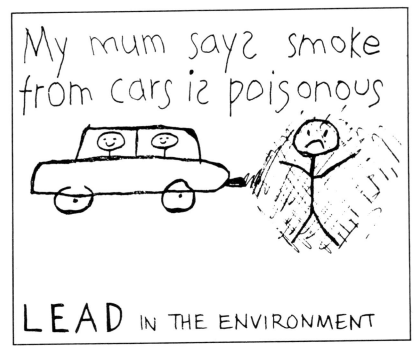

Fig. 1.4 Lead in the environment

varying amounts of lead in food which are not likely to constitute a serious risk at present but which are monitored continuously. Food and water, however, are only two of the possible sources of lead intake to the body. Concern today is also centred on the risk of high blood levels from lead pollution of the air and from some aspects of the home environment of the child. High levels of lead in the air, and the solid settling out as dust, may arise from specific industrial processes such as lead smelting and lead waste reclamation plants and from the exhaust fumes of petrol containing lead. In addition to existing restrictions, it is probable that the Government will eventually ban lead from petrol completely. Continuous monitoring of the lead content of the air and dust in large industrial areas is carried out regularly.

One of the main sources of lead in the home is old paint with a high lead content. Modern paint is required to be lead-free but many old houses, particularly those in multiple occupation, may have remained unpainted for years or have new paint superimposed on layers of old lead-containing paint. Some children living in these houses will pick off flaking paint and so run the risk of ingesting considerable amounts of lead. This is a particular risk in the very young, whose hand-to-mouth activities are common, and in older children with the habit (pica) of eating non-food substances such as paint and soil. Some houses are built on land containing industrial waste with a high lead content and the soil in play areas adjacent to the home may be contaminated.

The cultures of some Asian families have, at times, produced a special lead hazard in the use of Surma, an eye cosmetic with a high lead sulphide content. The Surma is applied to the edge of the eyelids from a very early age, in both boys and girls, to make their appearance more attractive. Some of it tends to be washed into the eyes and thence into the nose and throat, resulting in small daily accumulations of lead in the body. Another more recent source of lead for Asian children was in the sale (now banned) in Asian food shops of Bal Jival Chemco Baby Tonic, claimed to be of value to 'Children's Diseases, viz. variola, capillary bronchitis, greenish diarrhoea, rickets, coughs, convulsions'. The 'tonic' consisted of a spoon containing a solid brown material intended to be mixed with milk or water. The spoon had a lead content of 83.3 % and the filling also contained a lead compound.

Lead poisoning In children, lead poisoning may present with anorexia and, at times, other abdominal symptoms such as constipation, vomiting and colic. Anaemia is common and there may be decreased play activity. It is also claimed that high blood levels, albeit with none of the overt signs of lead poisoning, can lead to hyperactivity, lowered levels of intelligence and under-achievement at school. Clinical tests to confirm abnormally high lead intake include estimation of blood lead levels, detection of basophil stippling of red blood cells and X-ray of the long bones which show lines of increased density at the metaphysis. A careful investigation of the child's environment is then necessary to identify the source of the lead.

Treatment: This includes calcium edetate (EDTA) therapy and/or penicillamine therapy to remove the lead from the body cells. Anaemia is corrected by appropriate iron therapy. Removal of the environmental lead hazard is essential if the child is not to suffer from repeated lead poisoning. This is particularly important when lead-containing paint is the cause, and total stripping of domestic paint-work and re-decorating with lead-free paint is indicated.

Lead may be a hazard:

1   In old houses painted with old lead-containing paint
2   In the air from industrial processes and exhaust fumes
3   Occasionally in water

The environment of a child

1   Intra-uterine: maternal health
                    diet
                    freedom from infection
                    healthy social habits
2   Home: parents
           family size
           family income
           housing
3   The outside world: food
                        water
                        air

The future

We are seeing today in the overall health and well-being of the majority of children some of the results to which improved environmental conditions over the past years have contributed a great deal.

For the well-being of future generations it is essential that there is continuous review of the environment in which children grow, so that predictable hazards can be forestalled and unforeseen ones dealt with expeditiously. At the same time as recognising the happy results of change for many children, this should serve to bring into sharp relief the minority groups of children for whom conditions are still by no means as good as one would wish. Consideration can be given to programmes of positive discrimination, which will enable them to experience a basic environment in which full growth and development can take place.

2

Prevention of Communicable Disease

Organisms of all kinds—bacteria, viruses, protozoa and fungi—form part of the environment of children and their families. Many are harmless; with some, a balance has been achieved so that under normal circumstances they do not cause serious concern; others, however, commonly give rise to infections which constitute a large proportion of childhood illness. These vary in severity from the relatively mild conditions such as the common cold and chickenpox to the more serious ones such as whooping cough and meningitis.

Communicable diseases may be classified according to the way in which the causative organisms gain access into the body:

1 Air-borne or droplet transmission: the organism is inhaled.
2 Water-borne and food-borne transmission: the organism is ingested.
3 Direct contact transmission: the organism passes from body surface to body surface.
4 Transmission from animals and insects.

Air-borne or droplet transmission

The organisms suspended on small droplets of moisture are expelled from the mouth, pharynx or upper respiratory tract of an already infected person during ordinary breathing and talking and, to an even greater extent, by coughing and sneezing. The infected droplets may then be inhaled by another person and so gain entry into their air passages. Sometimes the organisms pass into the dust in rooms, and may remain there for a considerable time, capable of causing infection if the dust is inhaled. Many of the communicable diseases of childhood are transmitted by droplet infection, including the common cold, chickenpox, measles, whooping cough, mumps, rubella, viral and bacterial meningitis.

Water-borne and food-borne transmission

This is the method of transmission of pathogenic organisms inhabiting the intestinal tract of an infected person and excreted in the faeces. Although the title 'water-borne' implies spread through polluted drinking water, this is no longer a very apt description relevant to this country, at least, although it serves as a reminder of the necessity to maintain the purifying of supplies. The description 'food-borne', however, remains very important. Organisms excreted in the faeces of the infected person contaminate the hands as a result of faulty personal hygiene, particularly through neglect in washing the hands after using the toilet and before preparing food. The organisms may then be transferred from the hands to food and so reach the intestinal tract of another person. In the case of young children, play with toys handled by an infected child, inadequate cleansing of potties and lavatory seats, and the use of communal towels may also spread the infection. Examples of diseases transmitted in this way are gastro-enteritis, dysentery, infective hepatitis, typhoid and paratyphoid fevers.

Transmission by direct contact

Lesions caused by an infective organism on a body surface such as the skin and mucous membranes may be a source of infection to others by direct contact with the infected area. Impetigo, scabies and venereal diseases are transmitted in this way.

Transmission from animals and insects

Some communicable diseases are caused by organisms usually carried by animals or insects and which may enter the human body:

1 By direct contact with the animal e.g. ringworm in the hair of cats and dogs reaching the skin of children who stroke them.
2 Contact with soil or dust contaminated at some time by animal excreta e.g. tetanus, when the spores originally excreted in horse and cow dung may remain dormant in soil or street dust for long periods and contaminate wounds.
3 Deposition on food of organisms carried by flies from infected excreta e.g. salmonella (food poisoning).
4 Bites by animals or insects e.g. rabies and malaria.

Tranmission of infection

1 Air-borne or droplet
2 Water-borne and food-borne
3 Direct contact
4 From animals and insects

The following terms are often used in connection with communicable diseases:

Incubation period   When the organisms enter the body, by whatever route, there is usually a period of time during which they multiply and before clinical signs of illness become apparent. This is termed the incubation period, and varies with different infections from a few days to weeks. The entry of infective organisms into the body is, however, not invariably followed by the development of clinical infection. Much depends on the numbers of organisms, their virulence and the capacity of the individual to prevent their multiplication within the body (resistance).

The period of communicability   This is the length of time during which a person with a communicable disease remains a source of infection to other people.

A carrier   A person may harbour an infective organism in the body and not necessarily show signs of clinical illness, but may still be capable of passing on the organism to other people who may then develop the illness. This person is known as a carrier. Carrier states may develop with the typhoid bacillus (harboured in the intestine and gall-bladder), salmonella and dysentery bacilli (intestine), diphtheria bacillus (pharynx and nose), meningococcus (pharynx and nose) and haemolytic streptococcus (throat and nose).

Incidence   This refers to the number of cases of communicable disease occurring in an area.

Sporadic. Sometimes an isolated case may occur, the origin of which may be difficult to trace. This is termed a sporadic case.
Endemic. A communicable disease is said to be endemic when scattered cases predictably occur in an area from time to time.
Epidemic. This refers to many cases of the same communicable disease occurring in a locality within a short period of time.

Changes in incidence

The pattern of the incidence of some communicable diseases in this country has changed a great deal in the last century. A hundred years ago, epidemics of serious infection (for instance smallpox, cholera, diphtheria, scarlet fever, tuberculosis and typhoid fever) were common and occurred on a scale not encountered today. Not only were they responsible for many deaths in children, but very often the survivors were left with a legacy of chronic illness and handicap. Today, the picture is very different; some illnesses such as diphtheria and poliomyelitis have been almost completely eradicated, although the recent decline in the uptake of immunisation has increased the risk of their reappearance. The incidence of others has markedly declined, and deaths from, and complications of, communicable disease are correspondingly fewer. This improvement is the result of many factors:

Changes in organisms. Naturally occurring changes, as yet not fully understood, have taken place in the nature of some organisms, with the result that their effects are very much less severe. Scarlet fever, one of the conditions caused by the haemolytic streptococcus, has for some time appeared in a much milder form than in previous years.

Improved living conditions. Better standards of housing, smaller families, less overcrowding, adequate sanitation, pure water supplies, and measures to ensure the safety of milk and other foods have all reduced the risk of the spread of communicable disease. Malnutrition is less common. Most children today have a well-balanced diet, especially in regard to the protein, mineral and vitamin content, thus contributing to the build-up of the body's general resistance to infection.

Diagnosis and therapy. Early recognition of specific communicable disease is important in controlling its spread. Increasing knowledge, particularly about the nature of viruses, together with the wider availability of comprehensive and sensitive laboratory tests contributes to the prompt and accurate diagnosis of many communicable diseases. Modern therapy, which includes the use of anti-toxins, antibiotics, and sulphonamides has prevented death and many of the crippling complications, and has helped in the elimination of carrier states.

Control of spread. There has been a growing understanding of the ways in which communicable diseases are transmitted, and consequently the development of methods designed to limit their spread and to protect populations of susceptible people. These procedures remain of great importance if adequate control of communicable disease is to be maintained. They include:

1 Notification of communicable disease
2 Contact tracing
3 Special measures in nurseries and schools
4 Immunisation
5 Health education

Changes in incidence of communicable disease

1 Changes in organisms
2 Improved living conditions
3 Earlier diagnosis and therapy
4 Better control of spread

Notification of communicable disease

It is a legal requirement that the occurrence of the more serious communicable diseases be notified to the medical officer for environmental health (MOEH) known as the *proper officer*. The MOEH is a doctor designated for this purpose by the local authority, usually the district medical officer or a named specialist in community medicine. The MOEH works closely with the environmental health department of the local authority in the control of infection. Notification to the MOEH is the responsibility of the doctor first diagnosing the illness, whether this occurs in hospital or general practice, and a small fee is payable for this service. Once the MOEH is aware of a case of notifiable illness, he will then initiate action to limit the spread of the infection. This may include isolation of the patient and identification of the contacts.

The following diseases are notifiable:

Acute encephalitis
* Acute meningitis
* Acute poliomyelitis
Anthrax
Cholera
* Diphtheria
* Dysentery (amoebic
  and bacillary)
* Infective jaundice
Lassa fever
Leprosy
Leptospirosis
Malaria
Marburg disease
* Measles
* Ophthalmia neonatorum
Paratyphoid fever
Plague
Rabies
Relapsing fever
* Scarlet fever
Smallpox
* Tetanus
* Tuberculosis
Typhoid fever
Typhus fever
Viral haemorrhagic fever
* Whooping cough
Yellow fever

Although it is possible for a child to contract any infection, those marked * are of particular relevance in childhood.

Contact tracing

Anyone in contact with a person suffering from a communicable disease, or a carrier, may be at risk of developing the disease himself and passing it on to yet more people. When a case of notifiable illness occurs (e.g. poliomyelitis, diphtheria, tuberculosis or dysentery) it is important that contacts are traced so that general precautionary advice may be given and, in certain instances, movement amongst the public restricted or specific preventive treatment instituted (e.g. reinforcing doses of polio vaccine to close contacts). Tracing of contacts is usually carried out by the health visitor or the environmental health officer and is co-ordinated by the MOEH.

Special measures in schools and nurseries

A communicable disease may spread very rapidly from child to child when they are in close contact with each other, as in the day nursery or school classroom. Precautions have to be taken to ensure that an infectious child (whether the condition is notifiable or not) does not associate with the other children until the period of communicability is over. Guidelines are given as to the minimum period of exclusion recommended (Tables 2.1 and 2.2).

The MOEH and other community medical and nursing staff, work in close co-operation with the advisors in the local authority education and social services departments and with the staff of schools and day nurseries, so that a recognised procedure can be followed when a case of communicable disease arises. This includes advice about exclusion, surveillance of the other children, discussion on matters of general hygiene and specific measures such as disinfection of potties.

Immunity

The body is capable of dealing with infection in a general way through naturally occurring protective mechanisms present in the blood and tissues. For the young baby, breast milk is a good source of a complex protein substance (immunoglobulin A, IgA) which gives extra natural protection in the first months of life.

As well as this general natural immunity, additional protection against specific communicable diseases may be achieved in other ways.

Exposure to infection

Exposure to organisms causing a specific communicable disease in many instances results in protection against subsequent attack. In response to the primary attack of invading organisms, the body forms protective substances, specific for each condition, known as *antibodies*, which can be rapidly reinforced in any succeeding exposure. The duration of immunity produced in this way varies; fortunately, for many of the childhood infections (apart from the common cold) protection is long-lasting and second attacks, although not unknown, are rare.

Table 2.1 Inclusion and exclusion periods for the commoner communicable diseases

Disease	Normal Incubation Period (in days)	Period of communicability	Minimal Period of Exclusion	
			Cases (subject to clinical recovery)	Contacts
Bacillary Dysentery	1–7	Whilst organism is present in stools	Until clinically fit and, when necessary, bacteriological examination is clear	Siblings from primary or nursery schools should be excluded until bacteriological examination is clear
Chickenpox	14–21	From 1 day before to 6 days after appearance of rash	6 days from onset of rash	None
Diphtheria	2–5	Whilst the organism is present in nose or throat	Until bacteriological examination is clear	Until bacteriological examination is clear
Food Poisoning (including) Salmonellosis	2–48 hours according to cause	Varies according to cause	Until clinically fit and, when necessary, bacteriological examination is clear	None
German Measles (Rubella)	14–21	From a few days before to 4 days after onset of rash	4 days from onset of rash	None
Hepatitis A	15–50 (commonly 28)	From 1–2 weeks before to 1 week after onset	7 days from onset of jaundice	None
Measles	10–15 commonly 12 to onset of illness and 16 to appearance of rash	From a few days before to 7 days after onset of rash	7 days from onset of rash	None

Table 2.1 (*contd.*)

Disease	Normal Incubation Period (in days)	Period of communicability	Minimal Period of Exclusion	
			Cases (subject to clinical recovery)	Contacts
Meningococcal infection (Meningitis)	2–10 (commonly 2–5)	Whilst organism is present in nasopharynx	Until clinical recovery	None
Mumps	18–21	From 7 days before onset of symptoms to subsidence of swelling	Until swelling has subsided (7 days minimum)	None
Poliomyelitis	3–21	Whilst virus is present in stools	At the discretion of the Medical Officer for Environmental Health	At the discretion of the Medical Officer for Environmental Health
Streptococcal Infection	2–5	Whilst organism is present in nasopharynx	Until clinical recovery	None
Tuberculosis (Primary)	4–6 weeks		At the discretion of the physician	
Tuberculosis (Secondary)	variable	Whilst organism is present in sputum	Until declared to be non-infectious	None
Typhoid fever Paratyphoid fever	7–21 (usually 14) 1–10	Whilst organism is present in stools or urine	Until bacteriological examination is clear	None except for home contact
Whooping cough (Pertussis)	7–10	From 7 days after exposure to 21 days after onset of paroxysmal cough	21 days from onset of paroxysmal cough	None

Table 2.2   Exclusion periods of the commoner skin infections

Disease	Minimal Period of Exclusion
Impetigo	Until the skin is healed
Pediculosis	Until treatment has been received
Verrucae Plantaris (Plantar Warts)	Exclusion unnecessary provided the warts remain covered with occlusive plaster
Tinea Capitis (Ringworm of scalp)	Until cured
Tinea Corporis (Ringworm of body)	Exclusion not normally necessary during treatment unless evidence of epidemic
Ringworm of feet (athlete's foot)	Exclusion from barefoot activities unnecessary but treatment always advisable
Scabies	Exclusion unnecessary once adequate treatment of the child instituted

Active immunisation

Some communicable diseases are so serious that reliance on exposure to infection as a method of producing subsequent long-lasting immunity is not justifiable. Active immunisation enables the body to build up specific antibodies against some of the more serious communicable diseases in the same way as exposure to actual infection, but without the risks inherent in the naturally occurring illness. The conditions most likely to be of consequence in childhood, and for which immunisation is advised as a routine preventive measure, are:

Diphtheria	Measles
Whooping cough	Tuberculosis
Tetanus	Rubella
Poliomyelitis	

The routine vaccination of children against smallpox was discontinued in 1971 and this procedure will be carried out only if stipulated as a requirement for travel to certain foreign countries. A planned programme of immunisation (Table 2.3) ensures for each child primary protection against these conditions at the age of greatest vulnerability. The immunity generally takes a few weeks to develop fully and in the case of diphtheria, whooping cough, tetanus and polio 'booster' doses of the immunising agent are needed at subsequent ages to ensure continuing immunity.

The District Health Authority has the responsibility of maintaining recommended programmes of immunisation. The procedure itself may be carried out by the child's general practitioner (with the exception of BCG which is the responsibility of the school health service) or through the community child health services. Recent circulars from the Department of Health give guidance as to the extent to which nurses may, subject to appropriate training and adequate legal cover, be involved in immunising procedures.

Reactions All immunisations carry a slight possibility of untoward reactions occurring but before any procedure is recommended, whether in general or for an individual child, the need for protection will have been considered greatly to outweigh any risk. Modern methods of production ensure vaccines of a high degree of purity, and observance of general and specific contra-indications to immunisation greatly reduces the likelihood of severe reactions. A child should not be immunised if any of the following general contra-indications apply:

1   Illness or recovery from an illness.
2   A severe reaction to a preceding immunising procedure.
3   If vaccines containing live organisms (e.g. polio vaccine, BCG, and rubella vaccine) are required, these should not be given within one month of each other unless there are special indications for this as, for example, crash-courses in cases of urgent visits abroad.
4   Certain chronic illnesses, in particular, malignant conditions such as leukaemia or those where cortico-steroid therapy is being given.

Specific contra-indications to particular immunising agents will be mentioned when the relevant communicable disease is discussed. The advisability of identifying contra-indications in a particular child emphasises the need for accurate information about the medical history before immunisation is carried out.

Local reactions are fairly common. They appear at the site of the injection and take the form of varying degrees of redness and swelling of the surrounding tissue. The reaction is usually very temporary and will subside spontaneously without any intervention.

General reaction in a child may show as extreme irritability, unusually prolonged crying, refusal of feeds or undue lethargy and, very occasionally, collapse. If, following the administration of a vaccine, the child collapses with these symptoms, intramuscular adrenaline should be

Table 2.3 Schedule of vaccination and immunisation procedures

Age	Vaccine	Interval	Notes
During the first year of life	Triple vaccine (Diph/Tet/Pert/Vac/Ads*) and oral polio vaccine, 3 doses	2nd dose preferably after 6–8 weeks. 3rd dose preferably after 4–6 months	The first dose of triple vaccine, together with oral polio vaccine, should be given at the age of 3 months. If whooping cough is prevalent, an alternative course of triple vaccine with a month's interval between doses may be used. Such a course should be followed at 12–18 months by a dose of DT/Vac/Ads*. If pertussis vaccine is contra-indicated or declined by parents, diphtheria/tetanus vaccine (DT/Vac/Ads*) should be given. Unvaccinated parents should be given oral polio vaccine at the same time as their baby
During the second year of life	Measles vaccine	Not less than 3 weeks following another vaccine	The following groups are at special risk: 1 Children of one year upwards in residential care, entering nursery school or other day care establishment 2 Children with serious physical incapacity who are likely to develop severe illness as a result of natural measles infection. Contra-indications to vaccination should be observed, especially in immune-deficient states

At entry to school or nursery school	DT/Vac/Ads* and oral polio vaccine	Preferably at least 3 years after completing the basic course	
Between the 10th and 14th birthdays	BCG vaccine	Not less than 3 weeks between BCG and rubella vaccinations	For tuberculin-negative children, and tuberculin-negative contacts of any age (e.g. certain immigrant families)
Between the 10th and 14th birthdays	Rubella vaccine (girls only)	Not less than 3 weeks between BCG and rubella vaccinations	All girls of this age should be offered rubella vaccination, whether or not there is a past history of a rubella attack. Vaccination is also strongly recommended for adult women of child-bearing age who are sero-negative and susceptible. Warning to avoid pregnancy for 3 months after vaccination should be given, to avoid possible risk to the fetus
On leaving school, before employment or further education	Polio vaccine (oral or inactivated) and tetanus vaccine (Tet/Vac/Ads)		

*Ads = Adsorbed and refers to a special type of recommended vaccine given. Adrenaline and a 1 ml syringe and needle should always be readily available when immunising procedures are being carried out. It is important that a severe local reaction or any general reaction is reported to the child's doctor, both from the aspect of ensuring that no further injections of that particular immunising agent are given and the need to inform the Central Committee on the Safety of Drugs about untoward incidents.

Passive immunisation

The newly-born child receives temporary protection against common infections through the placental transfer of antibodies from the mother's blood. In the course of the first 5–6 months of life, this immunity gradually decreases in effectiveness but serves to give some protection to the child during the vulnerable period when his antibody-forming system has not yet fully developed.

Occasionally, immediate protection may be thought necessary if a child already suffering from some serious illness is exposed to an infection which would aggravate his original condition. An injection of human immunoglobulin (a part of the blood containing antibodies of many kinds) will either prevent the infection developing or lessen the severity of the attack. This protection has only a temporary life, as these antibodies are not generated by the child himself and so are eliminated from the body within a few weeks.

Ways of achieving immunity

1 Breast feeding
2 Exposure to infection
3 Active immunisation against diphtheria, tetanus, polio, whooping cough, measles, tuberculosis and rubella
4 Passive immunisation in special circumstances

Health education

Many people today are much more knowledgeable about communicable diseases but there is a continuing need for accurate information to enable the public to appreciate the common sense ways in which individuals may contribute to prevention and control. This is particularly relevant for parents of young children, and medical and nursing staff have a responsibility for promoting health education in this field by:

1 Giving factual information about common infections, their spread and simple methods of control.
2 Encouraging good standards of hygiene in the home, particularly in the preparation of milk feeds and the sterilisation of equipment.
3 Emphasising the importance of immunisation and encouraging use of the services available.

Methods of control

1 Notification of communicable disease
2 Contact tracing
3 Special measures in schools and nurseries
4 Immunisation
5 Health education

Some common communicable diseases in children

Chickenpox

Chickenpox is one of the most common infections in children, but is not regarded as a serious complaint, except in the very young baby.

Organism: The chickenpox virus

Transmission: Air-borne from a case

Incubation period: 14–21 days

Clinical picture: A characteristic rash appears within 24 hours of the onset of general malaise and moderate pyrexia. The rash starts as red spots on the chest and back with spread to the face, trunk and limbs. The spots become superficial vesicles which dry within 3–4 days forming scabs which eventually fall off and rarely leave a permanent scar. Successive crops of spots may arise for some days after the first eruption.

Treatment: The main difficulty is discomfort from the itching of the rash and attempts should be made to prevent scratching which may lead to secondary infection and scarring. Local soothing applications such as calamine lotion and a daily bath are helpful; nails should be kept short and cotton mittens can be worn during sleep.

Diphtheria

Diphtheria is an extremely serious condition, but fortunately rarely occurs in this country because of the efficacy of immunisation programmes.

Organism: The diphtheria bacillus

Transmission: Air-borne from a case or carrier

Incubation period: 2–5 days

Clinical picture: The early signs may give a misleading picture of the seriousness of the illness. The primary lesion is a greyish white tenacious membrane in the throat and/or nasal passages from which the diphtheria bacilli may be cultured. Sore throat is, however, not a prominent symptom. There is only a moderate pyrexia, but the child appears listless and lethargic, and the pulse rate may be raised. The main danger is from the effects of a powerful toxin produced by the diphtheria bacilli which may weaken the heart muscle and produce paralysis in other parts of the body, particularly the soft palate, muscles of the wrist and foot, and sometimes the diaphragm.

Treatment: Prompt isolation in hospital is essential, and diphtheria antitoxin is given without delay. Antibiotics are useful in preventing superimposed infection of the throat.

Prevention: Active immunisation of all young children is strongly advised. The primary course should ideally be completed by the end of the first year of life, and a 'booster' dose given at school entry. There are no specific contra-indications to diphtheria immunisation, although it is recommended that children over the age of 10 years should first have a preliminary skin test to establish the need for immunisation.

Gastro-enteritis

This is a term commonly used to describe diarrhoea and vomiting, which in babies and young children may be secondary to other conditions such as otitis media, but may also be caused by a primary infection of the alimentary tract. The infecting organism which is ingested in food, including milk feeds, could be one of many:

1 *Escherichia coli* (*E. Coli*) bacillus
2 Sonne dysentery bacillus
3 One of the *Salmonella* group of organisms
4 Viruses such as the Rota viruses and the Coxsackie virus
5 Protozoa

E. Coli. gastro-enteritis   This condition is one of the common intestinal infections in babies and young children and one of the most important. As well as the clinical cases, about 2% of apparently healthy young children excrete the organism in the faeces, and thus are a source of infection to others.

Transmission: Ingested in food

Incubation period: 1–5 days

Clinical picture: The illness may start as an acute episode of vomiting and diarrhoea with very fluid green stools, or it may develop in a more insidious manner. In young children, diarrhoea and vomiting of any degree of severity, and from whatever cause, should always be regarded as potentially serious and needing medical attention. Dehydration and disturbance of the blood chemistry may quickly occur, with potentially dangerous sequelae such as cerebral damage and sometimes death.

Treatment: Immediate treatment is aimed at preventing or remedying dehydration and maintaining the normal electrolyte balance of the blood by careful choice of fluid replacement. The use of antibiotics varies according to the sensitivity of the particular type of *E. Coli* found on stool culture.

Sonne dysentery   This form of gastro-enteritis is usually a mild infection although in small or frail babies it may have serious significance. The main trouble is its nuisance value as the infection tends to drag on over a period of time and, when occurring in children attending nurseries or school, may disrupt the normal routine.

Organism: Sonne dysentery bacillus (*Shigella sonnei*)

Incubation period: 3–7 days but may be of shorter duration

Transmission: Spread from infected faeces to the mouth of another person. Symptomless excreters of the dysentery bacillus are commonly found amongst the close contacts of a child with clinical symptoms.

Clinical picture: There is usually minimal general disturbance apart from mild pyrexia. The main presenting symptoms are abdominal pain and diarrhoea; vomiting is not common except in severe cases. In young children the stools are loose and green; in a few cases, small amounts of blood and mucus are present. The diarrhoea tends to decrease after 1–4 days.

Treatment: The Sonne dysentery bacillus varies widely in its response to sulphonamides and antibiotics, and sensitivity tests will indicate whether a particular drug is likely to be effective. Even without specific treatment, the infection gradually clears, but it may be up to 7–8 weeks before the organism ceases to be excreted. In the very young, dehydration and disturbance of electrolyte balance may need correction. Children attending day nurseries or nursery schools are excluded until 3 stool specimens taken at 3-day intervals are negative.

Prevention of infective gastro-enteritis   There is no specific immunising agent against gastro-enteritis caused by an infective organism. Prevention and control of spread relies on:

1   Scrupulous attention to hygiene when food is prepared, particularly cleanliness of the hands and nails, and for babies the adequate sterilisation of feeding utensils and equipment by boiling or chemical methods.
2   Protection of food from flies.
3   Where possible, refrigeration of food.
4   In schools and nurseries, exclusion of infected children, attention to adequate disinfection of potties, lavatory seats and handles, and use of individual towels are important preventive measures.

Infective hepatitis

Organism: Hepatitis A virus

Transmission: Food-borne from infected faeces

Incubation period: 15–50 days

Clinical picture: Infective hepatitis is an inflammatory condition of the liver, giving rise to anorexia, nausea with vomiting at times, and varying degrees of jaundice. In children it frequently takes a mild course with little or no jaundice apparent. There may be some tenderness beneath the right costal margin; the urine becomes dark from increased bile pigments, and the stools pale.

Treatment: There is no specific treatment for infective hepatitis. Confinement to bed is not invariably necessary and is largely regulated by the activity of the child himself. Similarly, restriction of diet is often self-selected—many children with this condition have a profound distaste for fatty food. Recovery is gradual but usually complete liver function returns.

Prevention: Spread of the virus is difficult to control but strict attention to personal hygiene offers the best chance of prevention. Immunoglobulin is of value for children in residential institutions.

Measles

Measles is a common infection in young children, and is usually relatively mild, although serious complications may occur in a proportion of children.

Organism: The measles virus

Transmission: Air-borne from a case

Incubation period: 10–15 days

Clinical picture: The early signs of measles may resemble a feverish cold—pyrexia, runny nose, cough and congestion of the conjunctiva. The rash comes on the fourth day after onset of symptoms, has a blotchy pinkish appearance, and starts on the face and behind the ears, spreading to the trunk. Measles is infectious *before* the rash appears and so the recognition of the significance of early signs is important. An aid to early diagnosis is the appearance of small white spots (Koplik's spots) on the mucous membrane of the mouth. Complications of measles include bronchopneumonia, otitis media and, less commonly, encephalitis.

Treatment: Antibiotics are usually reserved for the treatment of complications. General nursing care includes care of the eyes when conjunctivitis is marked

Prevention: Immunisation against measles is offered routinely to children in the second year of life and consists of a single injection. Special consideration should be given about the advisability of measles immunisation when there is a history of convulsions in the child, or of egg allergy. Fewer than 70 % of children in England and Wales are immunised against measles. In some children, when measles could be a grave threat to health, an injection of human immunoglobulin given within five days of exposure will prevent or modify the severity of the attack.

Meningitis

Meningitis is not a common infection of childhood but is one of the most dangerous.

Organism: Usually the meningococcus, but may also be the pneumococcus, or a virus. Tuberculous meningitis is now rare in this country.

Transmission: Air-borne from a case or carrier

Incubation period: 2–10 days

Clinical picture: Early diagnosis is important if treatment is to be effective but the symptoms are not always specific. The important symptoms are severe headache, vomiting, stiffness of the neck and back and, in a proportion of meningococcal infections, a pinkish-red rash, particularly on the body. Convulsions, diarrhoea and vomiting may be early symptoms in young children. Complications may include deafness and mental retardation.

Treatment: Hospital admission is essential. Treatment is with appropriate antibiotics and sulphonamides.

Prevention: No immunisation is available, but sulphonamide therapy for close contacts of an established case of meningococcal meningitis has been advocated.

Mumps

Mumps is usually a mild disease in children.

Organism: The mumps virus

Transmission: Air-borne

Incubation period: 18–21 days

Clinical picture: Mumps is primarily an infection of the salivary glands, in particular the parotid gland, where swelling gives rise to pain, stiffness and difficulty in chewing. Although not a severe illness in children, occasionally it is complicated in boys by inflammation of the testicles (orchitis) which could give rise to later sterility.

Treatment: There is no specific treatment; an easily managed diet and mouth washes may relieve discomfort and the difficulties of chewing.

Prevention: A vaccine against mumps is available but is not yet used routinely in this country.

Poliomyelitis

Poliomyelitis is now a rare condition in this country due to the success of immunisation procedures. Its continued absence is dependent on a high level of immunisation uptake.

Organism: One of the three types of polio virus

Transmission: Air-borne and water/food-borne

Incubation period: 3–21 days

Clinical picture: Poliomyelitis starts with the symptoms of a feverish cold—pyrexia, sore throat and aching limbs. In some children the illness progresses no further and its true nature may never be recognised. In others, the infection continues with severe pains in the limbs, headache, and stiffness of the neck and back. The illness may then subside, but a proportion of cases go on to flaccid paralysis of muscles, varying from a minimal involvement of small groups to wide-spread paralysis including the muscles of respiration. Death may occur from brain stem involvement and, in the survivors, there may be residual permanent handicap of differing severity.

Treatment: Early diagnosis and hospital admission are essential. Complete rest is an important feature of nursing care in an attempt to limit the spread of muscle involvement. Physiotherapy may later be needed to minimise the degree of residual handicap.

Prevention: Immunisation against poliomyelitis should be carried out in the first year of life with 'booster' doses on school entry and leaving. The vaccine is given orally and there are no specific contra-indications. Unvaccinated parents of a child who is being immunised should be given the oral vaccine at the same time. A prophylactic dose of vaccine is recommended for close contacts of an established case of poliomyelitis, even though an immunisation course has already been completed.

Rubella (German Measles)

Rubella is usually a very mild infection in children, so much so that occasionally it may almost pass unnoticed. The main area of concern is the effect on the developing fetus should the mother become infected in the early weeks of pregnancy. This gives a greatly increased risk of deafness, congenital cataract, heart defect and mental retardation in the baby.

Organism: Rubella virus

Transmission: Air-borne from a case

Incubation period: 14–21 days

Clinical picture: Rubella is characterised by a rash rather like that of measles in its distribution but less blotchy in appearance. The cervical and occipital glands are usually enlarged

Treatment: No specific treatment is indicated

Prevention: Immunisation against rubella is offered as a routine procedure (regardless of a history of previous rubella) to girls between their 10th and 14th birthdays so that they will be protected during the child-bearing period. Immunisation is also available to older girls and women in the child-bearing age group, but the procedure is more elaborate. A preliminary blood sample is tested for rubella antibodies and their absence indicates the need for immunisation. Pregnancy is an absolute contra-indication to rubella immunisation and reliable contraceptive measures should be taken for three months following immunisation. Screening for rubella antibodies forms part of the routine blood testing in the ante-natal period and, where indicated, immunisation can be given soon after the delivery.

Scarlet fever

In recent years, scarlet fever has become a much less severe condition than previously.

Organism: Haemolytic streptococcus

Transmission: Air-borne

Incubation period: 1—7 days

Clinical picture: Scarlet fever often has an abrupt onset with pyrexia, sore throat, vomiting and headache. The rash appears on the second day as bright red pin-point spots on the face and neck, rapidly involving the rest of the body. Although usually mild, it must be remembered that scarlet fever is just one of the manifestations of haemolytic streptococcal infection and complications such as chronic rheumatic heart disease, nephritis and otitis media may still occur.

Treatment: Penicillin G is the drug of choice in treatment of haemolytic streptococcal infection

Prevention: There are no specific preventive measures.

Tetanus

Tetanus is a dangerous condition which arises when cuts and wounds become contaminated with dust or soil containing the tetanus bacilli. It is a hazard associated with injury in road accidents and playing fields.

Incubation period: 7—14 days, but may be longer

Clinical picture: There may be a history of a wound, round which redness, tenderness and local muscle spasm develop. Pain and stiffness follow in the muscles of the face and neck, causing extreme difficulty in swallowing. Generalised muscle spasms develop and death may follow from heart failure and exhaustion.

Treatment: Hospitalisation is essential. Treatment includes neutralisation of the toxin produced by the tetanus bacilli with tetanus immunoglobulin, antibiotic therapy, muscle relaxants and sedation.

Prevention: Tetanus is effectively prevented by immunisation. This forms part of the routine immunisation schedule in the first years of life, with 'booster' doses at school entry and leaving. Any wound where contamination with tetanus bacilli is considered a possibility should be thoroughly cleaned. An injection of tetanus toxoid is given as a precautionary measure even if immunisation has been completed. If there has been no previous immunisation, the tetanus toxoid injection should be regarded as the first of a course to be completed subsequently. There are no specific contra-indications to tetanus immunisation, but it is recommended that repeated 'booster' doses, whether prophylactic or routine, should not be given within a year.

Tuberculosis

Tuberculous infection of children is now relatively rare due to the safety measures taken to ensure tubercle-free milk, BCG vaccination programmes, and the effect of chemotherapy in decreasing the numbers of infected people in the community. BCG vaccination is offered routinely to school children between the ages of 10 and 13 years when preliminary skin-testing indicates a lack of immunity.

In special circumstances, BCG may be given at any age from birth onwards; early vaccination is recommended for children at risk of exposure to a known infected person and for children born into immigrant households, where the likelihood of contact is greater than in the general population.

Whooping cough (pertussis)

Whooping cough is still regarded as a serious infection in that complications, sometimes fatal, may develop in a minority of children, particularly during the first year of life. Young babies are particularly at risk as they receive no passive immunity against whooping cough from their mother, and low rates of immunisation in the general child population increase the likelihood of transmission of infection from older siblings.

Organism: *Bordetella pertussis*—a cocco-bacillus

Transmission: Air-borne from a case

Incubation period: 7–10 days

Clinical picture: Whooping cough starts with symptoms similar to those of a cold, followed by the development of a paroxysmal cough, the prolonged spasms ending in a typical 'whoop'. Vomiting at the end of the coughing episode is common and may lead to considerable weight loss. The condition is very distressing for child and parent, and the cough tends to continue for some time after the infection has ceased. Complications are bronchopneumonia, chronic bronchiectasis and, more rarely, encephalitis. Admission to hospital is recommended for young babies, who may develop episodes of apnoea following a spasm of coughing.

Treatment: Once the symptoms are well-established, antibiotics have little effect on the infection itself, but a course of erythromycin given in the early stages may reduce the risk of respiratory tract complications. General treatment includes sedatives and careful attention to dietary intake—it may be necessary, when vomiting is troublesome, to give frequent small feeds in the intervals between paroxysms of coughing.

Prevention: Immunisation against whooping cough is offered in the first year of life, and is usually given as part of the 'triple' vaccine containing diphtheria and tetanus toxoids, together with pertussis vaccine.

In the past few years, considerable debate has taken place and publicity been given to the allegation that a small number of children developed permanent brain damage following whooping cough immunisation. Detailed investigations have been made by the Joint Committee on Vaccination and Immunisation and include the findings of the National Childhood Encephalopathy Study published in 1980, which estimated the risk of persistent neurological damage following whooping cough immunisation to be in the order of 1 in 100 000. This is considered to be a very small risk compared with the benefits of immunisation against a serious infection of childhood. The DHSS has issued advice that the following contra-indications should be considered:

1 It is advisable to postpone vaccination if the child is suffering from any acute febrile illness, particularly respiratory, until fully re-covered (minor infections without fever or systemic upset are not regarded as a contra-indication).

2 Vaccination should not be carried out in children who have:

   (a) A history of any severe local or general reaction (including a neurological reaction) to a preceding dose

(b) A history of cerebral irritation or damage in the neonatal period, or who have suffered from fits or convulsions.

3 There are certain groups of children in whom whooping cough vaccination is not absolutely contra-indicated but who require special consideration as to its advisability. These groups are:

(a) Children whose parents or siblings have a history of idiopathic epilepsy.
(b) Children with developmental delay thought to be due to a neurological defect.
(c) Children with neurological disease.

For these groups the risk of vaccination may be higher than in normal children but the effects of whooping cough may be more severe, so that the benefits of vaccination would also be greater. The balance of risk and benefit should be assessed with special care in each individual case, and the advice of a paediatrician or paediatric neurologist sought if necessary.

A personal or family history of allergy has, in the past, been regarded as a contra-indication to vaccination but there is now a substantial body of medical opinion which no longer considers this to be so. Doctors should, however, use their own discretion in each individual case.

Even when pertussis vaccine is contra-indicated an infant should still be considered for immunisation against diphtheria and tetanus.

Parents should be asked to discuss specific questions prior to immunisation (Table 2.4).

Skin infections in children

Impetigo

Organism: Usually staphylococcus or streptococcus

Transmission: Direct contact by touching a lesion, or spread through use of communal towels

Clinical picture: Impetigo begins with red spots appearing most commonly on the face or hands. The spots become encrusted and irritating and may spread rapidly, especially if the lesions are rubbed or scratched. Because of its contagious nature, exclusion from school or nursery is recommended until healing has taken place.

Treatment: Local application of antibiotic creams is usually effective.

Table 2.4 A card given to parents prior to immunisation of their child

IMMUNISATION

Please read the following questions before your Child is Immunised

1. Has your Child had any convulsions (fits) at any time?
2. Has anyone in the family had convulsions?
3. Was your Child unwell during the new-born period?
4. Is your Child unwell today?
5. Is he/she receiving medicine prescribed by your doctor?
6. If your Child has already started the course of immunisation, was he/she unwell after the first or second injection?
7. Has your Child shown signs of an allergy?

If the ANSWER to any of these questions is YES, or if you are not sure, tell the Clinic Doctor BEFORE an injection is given.

Scabies

Organism: The scabies mite

Transmission: Close contact with an infected person or clothes and sheets used by them

Clinical picture: The scabies mite burrows under the skin, particularly in the web of the fingers, the wrist and the elbow. Intense irritation, especially at night, is caused; scabies is perhaps the commonest cause of generalised itching. Scratching can lead to secondary infection. The diagnosis is established by identification of the characteristic burrow showing as a thread-like elevation on the skin surface.

Treatment: It is very important that the whole family is treated, not just the infected child, otherwise recurrence is almost inevitable. The treatment consists of the application on two successive days of 25 % benzyl benzoate emulsion to the whole body—no area should be left untreated. Once treatment has been instituted, exclusion from school is unnecessary.

Head lice

The number of children with head lice appears to be rising. This may be due to changing fashions of hair style and care and the resistance of lice to methods of treatment.

Transmission: Lice can easily wander from person to person when heads are in close proximity.

Clinical picture: The common way by which infestation is detected is the recognition of the pearly grey eggs (nits) on the hair. The nits adhere very firmly to the hair, and severe itching and secondary infection may result.

Treatment: Malathion preparations such as Prioderm, are freely applied to the scalp, followed in 24 hours by shampooing and thorough combing of the hair. Infestation is usually a family condition. The home should be visited by the health visitor or school nurse and treatment offered to the other members of the family. The child should be excluded from school until treated.

Plantar warts (verrucae)

Warts on the sole of the foot, as on other parts of the body, are caused by a virus infection. Plantar warts are contagious and the infection may be picked up by the child walking barefoot in swimming baths or gymnasia.

Treatment: Various methods of treatment have been tried, including soaking the wart in formalin, scraping, and the application of wart-removing paints or medicated discs. Exclusion from school is not indicated, provided the verruca is kept covered, but the child should not go to the swimming baths unless the foot can be kept fully covered as by the wearing of special plastic socks.

Present achievements and problems

Communicable disease in children presents an ever-changing series of situations and challenges.

Programmes of immunisation have resulted in spectacular decreases in the incidence of diphtheria and poliomyelitis (Fig. 2.1) and deaths due to these conditions. With measles, whooping cough (Fig. 2.2) and tuberculosis there is no doubt that immunisation has played a big part in the improved situation, but in these conditions there are also other important contributory factors such as chemotherapy and antibiotics, better nutrition and housing. The effect of rubella immunisation on the

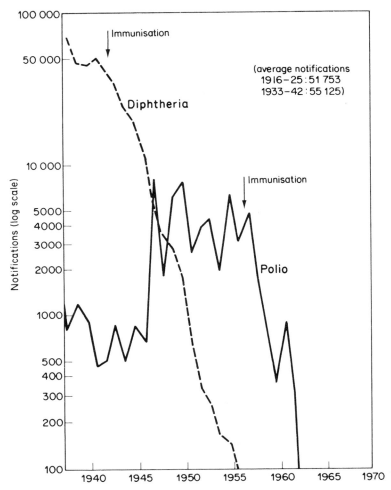

Fig. 2.1 Poliomyelitis and diphtheria notifications 1940–70 (England and Wales)

incidence of congenital malformations is in process of evaluation.

If recurrence of infections such as diphtheria and poliomyelitis is to be prevented, it is very important that high levels of immunisation are maintained in the child population. The debate on the safety of whooping cough immunisation has aroused anxiety in parents to the extent that, in some instances, all immunisations have been refused. Parents need consistent advice from medical and nursing staff, and continued support to enable them to decide wisely on issues which they

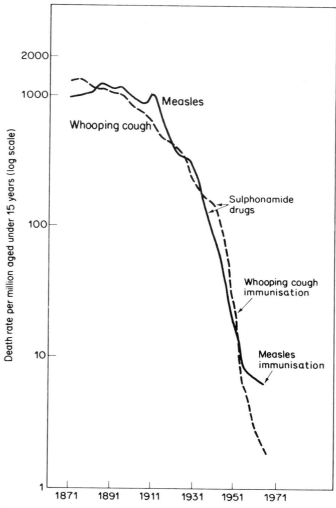

Fig. 2.2 Childhood mortality from measles and whooping cough 1871–1971
(England and Wales)

realise may affect the health and happiness of their child.

Not all communicable diseases are preventable by immunisation; this is particularly true of many of the virus infections. It is hoped that in the foreseeable future vaccines will become available for protection against rota viruses, infective hepatitis and cytomegalic virus infection which, if occurring during pregnancy, is thought to be an even more important cause than rubella of mental retardation in the child.

Many families today holiday abroad in countries where communicable diseases still present a considerable health hazard, and there is a risk of conditions such as typhoid fever, cholera and poliomyelitis being contracted abroad and brought back into this country. This widens our concern, not only on behalf of children resident here, but those growing up in the under-developed countries.

3
Indices of Health

A profile of child health in the country as a whole, and its constituent regions and districts, illustrates the extent to which services are helping to achieve the full potential for health and development, and assists in efficient planning for the future. Such a composite picture can be drawn from statistical information about the total number of children in each age group and the pattern of their lives—birth, growth and development, social environment and, in some cases, illness, accident, handicap or death. These statistics are derived from numerical facts, systematically collected and relating to data from large numbers of children. Individual hospital and community workers are usually involved with comparatively small numbers of children. Consequently, they may form a subjective impression of collective health or ill-health which, although very valuable within its own limits, is not necessarily true of the majority of children. The use of statistics helps to redress the balance and enables an assessment to be made of the changes required to meet the common health needs of all children and the special needs of particular groups such as the handicapped.

Sources of information

At different times in history, more especially during the last two centuries, measures have been introduced to provide accurate data about children, their health and related social and educational circumstances. Information is now collected and presented for each administrative level in the health service—district, regional and national. At national level, the Office of Population Censuses and Surveys (OPCS)—formerly known as the General Register Office—receives information from local sources and subsequently issues at regular intervals statistics relevant to the whole country and its regions and districts. Thus a picture of child health is presented which enables comparisons to be made both in a historical sense, comparing different centuries, decades and years, and geographically, examining similarities and differences in statistics for other countries, regions and districts. An annual report is also published by the Chief Medical Officer of the Department of Health, setting out 'The State of the Public Health' and including references to particular aspects of child health.

The chief sources of information are:

1 The census The census provides factual information about the total population of the country. It was first introduced in 1801 and, with the

exception of 1941, has continued at 10 yearly intervals. Great organis-
ational care is taken to ensure maximum accuracy. The census enables
numerical data to be compiled about:

(a) The number of people in the country, their age and sex.
(b) Marital status.
(c) Birthplace, nationality and country of origin.
(d) Occupation.

It thus provides social information which links up closely with the health
and well-being of children—family size, social class and the numbers of
children in one parent families. The census is also used to plan services of
different kinds for years ahead, and information is obtained about
environmental factors such as housing. Based on the 1981 census, the
estimated mid-year population of England and Wales was 49 592 900, of
whom 10 118 600 were aged 14 years and under.

2 Registration procedures The law requires that:

(a) All births (live and still-births) are to be registered with the local
     registrar of births, marriages and deaths within 42 days of the child
     being born. The responsibility for registration lies with the parents
     of the child, who then receive the birth certificate or certificate for
     burial of a still-born child.
(b) All deaths are to be registered with the local registrar within five
     days of the event. No burial or cremation can take place until a
     disposal order has been obtained from the registrar or a coroner's
     order issued.

The number of births and deaths registered each year is used to
calculate:

Birth rate: the number of live births occurring in any year per 1000
population
Still-birth rate: the number of still-births occurring in any year per 1000
total (live and still) births
Illegitimate births: expressed as a percentage of the total live births
Death rate: the number of people dying in any year per 1000 population
Infant Mortality rate: the number of children in any year dying in the
first year of life per 1000 live births.

Registration of births and deaths also enable population figures to be
adjusted annually.

3 Notification of births Every birth (live and still) must be notified by
the midwife or doctor to the District Medical Officer within 36 hours of
the birth taking place. On receipt of the birth notification, the child's
health record can then be started. In some districts the birth notification

forms the beginning of a computerised record but, whatever the procedure, the appropriate health visitor is made aware of the birth of the child.

In some respects, notification and registration of births may appear to be a duplication of effort. The reason for two procedures lies in the historical background, and is still very relevant today. Registration of births became a legal requirement in 1836 and preceded notification by many years. It was realised that much earlier knowledge of the child's existence was needed to enable health visitor supervision to be commenced early enough to safeguard the health and welfare of the child in the very vulnerable first few weeks of life, and so notification within 36 hours of birth became legal in 1915. The birth notification form also provides information of clinical and statistical value which is not available from registration sources, such as the birth weight, period of gestation and presence of congenital anomaly.

4 Information on illness and handicap   Through the registration and notification procedures it is possible to obtain information on virtually all births and deaths. Where other conditions such as non-fatal illness, accident or later handicap are concerned, comparable information is patchy. The following sources of information give part, but not all, of the picture:

Notification of congenital abnormality. Initial identification of a baby born with a congenital abnormality appears on the birth notification form. The District Medical Officer is then required to make a monthly return to the OPCS giving more detailed information on all babies both live and still-born with any congenital defect whatever the degree of severity. This procedure provides a picture of the national and local incidence of specific defects, and constitutes an 'early warning' system of any gross departure from the expected pattern needing further investigation.

Hospital activity analysis. Some information about the incidence of illness in children is obtained through hospital activity analysis (HAA) which gives details about the number of children admitted to hospital, the condition diagnosed and the length of stay. There is, as yet, no comparable analysis of attendance at out-patient clinics and accident and emergency departments, although the Royal College of General Practitioners has, from time to time, undertaken surveys of medical consultation and hospital admission rates from within general practice.

Notification of communicable diseases. Some of the more serious communicable diseases to which children may be particularly vulnerable are required by law to be notified to the proper officer (Chapter 2).

Notification of handicap. In many districts, a notification system of handicap in a child is in operation and a register is compiled of all children who have a substantial degree of handicap, particularly one which is likely to be permanent and need special services.

5 Statistical returns   Each district and region forward data to the Department of Health regarding community services for children, for example the number of children visited by the health visitors, child health clinic attendances, school health service examinations and uptake of immunisation. These statistics provide considerable information about the way in which preventive services available to all children are functioning and the extent to which they are being used.

6 National and local surveys   Available routine statistics do not always give sufficient detailed information about specific aspects of child health. From time to time national or local surveys are undertaken to examine in more depth some topics of interest or concern. Recent national surveys include the Study of Childhood Encephalopathy (which has special relevance to the incidence of cerebral damage following whooping cough immunisation), a long-term study of Malignant Disease in Childhood, the National Perinatal Mortality Study, the National Child Development Studies (which follow the progress of a cohort of children born in 1970) and the Multicentre Study of Infant Deaths.

Sources of statistical information

1 The Census
2 Registration of births and deaths
3 Notification of births
4 Notification of illness and handicap
5 Community child health statistical returns
6 National and local surveys

Statistical data has its place in consideration of all areas of child health, but the remainder of this chapter will be dealing mainly with the use of specific information relating to the first fundamental issue in the lives of children—the question of survival. It is perhaps paradoxical that for many years the traditional index of the health of children has been expressed in terms of death (the infant mortality rate). This, however, is understandable when considered against its historical background dating from the days when the struggle just to survive in the first year of life was an overwhelming priority.

The infant mortality rate (IMR)

This is defined as the number of children dying in any one year before the age of one, out of every 1000 live births.

Fig. 3.1 shows the trend in infant mortality rates and the spectacular decline since the beginning of the present century. This decrease has been the result of many interacting influences, which can be summarised in four broad categories:

1 Social factors Many social changes, particularly in the last 40–50 years, have contributed to the declining infant mortality rate. These include smaller families, financial benefits, improved nutrition and dietary supplements, and better housing conditions.

2 Improved ante-natal and perinatal care The Midwives Act (1902), in forbidding anyone to practise as a midwife without a recognised qualification, emphasised the need for a much higher standard of care for all women at the time of delivery. Since then, the maternity services

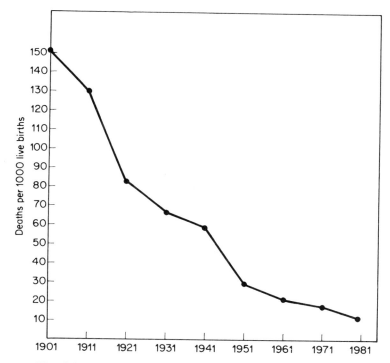

Fig. 3.1 Infant mortality (1901–1981) in England and Wales

have developed enormously. The increased availability of hospital delivery, improved training of professional staff and organisation of ante-natal care, including health education, have played an important part in reducing the IMR, particularly in its first-week-deaths component.

3   Advances in medical care   Within the last 50 years or so the outlook for many serious and potentially lethal or handicapping illnesses in childhood has completely changed, owing to the introduction of immunising agents, antibiotics and other modern therapeutic drugs, and advances in biochemical techniques which enable the blood chemistry of children to be monitored and maintained in balance.

4   Health services   The present century has seen the rapid growth of health services focused on the special needs of children, both in the preventive and curative fields.

Improvement of infant mortality

1   Better ante-natal and perinatal care
2   Advances in medical care
3   Improved social conditions
4   Development of health services

In 1981 the infant mortality rate for England and Wales was 11.1, the lowest since records began. The chief causes of death in children under the age of one year were:

1   Congenital anomalies
2   Anoxic conditions
3   Respiratory diseases
4   Sudden death (cause unknown).

Facts and figures, however, are of limited value unless used constructively. Improved though the IMR may be, there still remains the feeling that even 12 or 13 children dying out of every 1000 born alive are too many, especially since rates in other comparable countries are lower. In considering infant mortality statistics, it is important to ask what further can be done to prevent death occurring, and to go beyond this and ask whether the measures taken to prevent death will also ensure a better quality of life for the survivors. Used in this way, a negatively charged statistic such as death can be the starting point for positive action for healthy survival.

It is useful, at this point, to break down the first year of life into two periods:

1 *The perinatal period,* covering the time of birth and the first week of life (the early neonatal period)
2 *The post-perinatal period,* from one week to one year.

The perinatal period

In considering the well-being of babies in the perinatal period, there are two main areas for concern:

1 The perinatal mortality rate
2 The health of the survivors, particularly those in the high-risk groups, where events at birth or in the first week of life could have implications for future well-being.

Perinatal mortality rate

This is defined as the number of still-births occurring in any one year plus the number of infants dying in the first week of life during that year per 1000 total (live and still) births. Still-births and first-week deaths are grouped together for this purpose because it is recognised that, for the most part, similar underlying factors are operative in both categories.

Figure 3.2 shows the steady decline in perinatal mortality rates in England and Wales since 1928 (the first year in which this rate was calculated). The rate in 1981 was 11.8. The chief clinical conditions associated with perinatal death are low birth weight, congenital abnormality, and hypoxia.

Improvement of perinatal mortality

It is recognised that the successful outcome of pregnancy is influenced not only by the quality of obstetric care but also by factors associated with the mother herself (Fig. 3.3), such as social class, ethnic group, and her attitude to the use of health and social services.

1 Social influences Important though the ante-natal period is, the early foundations for a healthy infant can be established long before pregnancy begins by trying to ensure the good health of the mother at the time of conception. Community child health staff, particularly school doctors, health visitors and the school nurses, have an important role to play in encouraging positive attitudes to health in school and college years. They must stress the value of a good diet with practical suggestions for times of economy and financial hardship, underline the potential harm caused by smoking and excessive alcohol, and explain

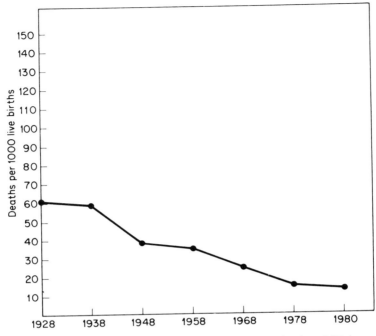

Fig. 3.2 Perinatal mortality (1928–1978) in England and Wales

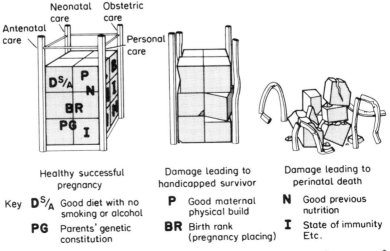

| Healthy successful pregnancy | Damage leading to handicapped survivor | Damage leading to perinatal death |

Key **D^S/$_A$** Good diet with no smoking or alcohol

PG Parents' genetic constitution

P Good maternal physical build

BR Birth rank (pregnancy placing)

N Good previous nutrition

I State of immunity Etc.

Fig. 3.3 Inter-relationship of factors leading to successful and unsuccessful pregnancy outcome

the available services and their sensible use (particularly rubella immunisation programmes, family planning and maternity services). Many family planning clinics give pre-conception advice when pregnancy is contemplated.

The ante-natal period itself should be regarded as a time for planned preventive health, with co-ordination of effort amongst all professionals who have a responsibility for some aspect of care. The health visitor and midwife, working closely together, can advise early and regular attendance for ante-natal supervision and reinforce earlier health education regarding diet, social habits and preparation for breast-feeding. It is particularly important to seek out and actively encourage those women who may already be at a disadvantage socially rather than wait for the initial approach to come from them—in many instances too late for preventive measures to have their full effect. This entails some precise explanation of the benefits of early care, by way of incentive, and helping the woman to assume some degree of responsibility for her own ante-natal health rather than total reliance on other agencies.

2 Ante-natal care Supervision during the ante-natal period is ideally a carefully planned and co-ordinated procedure undertaken by hospital obstetric staff, general practitioner and midwife. It involves an assessment of the woman herself and her social background, monitoring of progress (particularly of maternal health and the growth of the fetus *in utero*), recognition of possible risks and, where indicated, planned intervention. Certain early screening procedures which have a direct bearing on fetal well-being are essential to reduce the risk of perinatal death and handicap.

(a) Blood examination
Haemoglobin estimation may indicate anaemia which is often associated with nutritional deficiency.

Serological tests for sexually transmitted diseases in the mother enable conditions potentially harmful to the infant, such as syphilis, to be treated effectively.

Blood grouping includes identification of the Rhesus factor. About 83 % of people in this country are Rhesus positive, the remaining 17 % Rhesus negative. When a woman is found to be Rhesus negative, further tests are advisable during pregnancy to exclude any incompatibility between her Rhesus negative blood and the blood of her baby which could result in severe degrees of anaemia and jaundice in the baby (i.e. haemolytic disease of the newborn). Rhesus incompatibility was first recognised in 1939–40. Since then, advances in the treatment of an affected baby and the prevention of incompatibility developing have resulted in haemolytic disease of the newborn as a cause of perinatal mortality and morbidity gradually disappearing.

Rubella antibody estimation should form part of the routine early ante-natal examination to establish whether the mother possesses adequate immunity to rubella. If not, advice is given about avoiding contact with cases of rubella, particularly in the early weeks of pregnancy, and arrangements are made for immunisation immediately after delivery to ensure future protection.

(b) Screening for fetal abnormality
A few serious defects in the developing baby may be diagnosed or strongly suspected by tests carried out in the early stages of pregnancy. The two most important investigations are:

Examination of maternal blood to estimate the amount of a substance known as alpha-feto-protein (AFP). This may be greatly increased when the developing baby has a severe defect of the central nervous system, such as spina bifida. When the result is suspiciously high, this is followed by an examination of AFP in the amniotic fluid. If this is also at a high level, it would confirm the presence in the fetus of a severe defect of the nervous system.

Chromosome analysis of the fetal cells in the amniotic fluid will detect Down's syndrome (Mongolism). The test should be available to pregnant women over the age of 35 years, or those who already have a child with a handicap due to a chromosome abnormality.

When either of these tests indicate that there is a strong possibility of abnormality, termination of pregnancy can be considered, thus preventing the birth of a seriously handicapped child.

3 Care at birth   The great majority of deliveries take place in hospital maternity units, and the few home deliveries are due more to the insistence of the parents rather than to lack of hospital facilities. Home delivery, however, as seen through the eyes of the expectant parents, is not always viewed with the same enthusiasm by the professional staff, though the common concern of all is for the safety of mother and child. Distance to travel for delivery, lack of familiar homely surroundings, fear of the unknown, dislike of feeling obliged to submit to hospital practices (such as shaving, conventional position for delivery, and episiotomy) are all factors which may influence attitudes to place of delivery and should be taken into account when reviewing hospital maternity services. One of the outstanding persuasive factors for hospital delivery is immediate skilled help being available should difficulties arise during or after the time of birth. Continuous monitoring of the progress of labour and the provision of sufficient numbers of special and intensive care baby units, with adequately trained medical and nursing staff, contribute to the reduction of deaths, particularly in the very low birth weight babies, those suffering from severe anoxia, and those needing surgical intervention.

4 Care of the newborn Not only is the first week of life important from the aspect of preventing death, but it should also be regarded as the start of life in a very positive way. Some happenings in this period may have implications for the quality of future survival:

Prevention of future handicap. Screening tests carried out in the first week of life for the detection of congenital dislocation of the hip, phenylketonuria and hypothyroidism are early preventive measures designed to prevent future handicap, and will be discussed in detail in the following chapters. Advances in other aspects of care of the newborn, particularly in the management of the very low birth weight babies and in the surgical treatment of some of the more serious abnormalities, result in babies remaining alive who in previous years would undoubtedly have died.

Mother-child relationship. The first few days of life are the time when the foundations of strong mother-child attachment (bonding) are laid down. Separation of mother and child during this period may lead to extreme maternal anxiety, lack of self-confidence, feeding difficulties, inability to experience fully the expected and long-awaited feelings of warmth towards the child, and even to rejection and non-accidental injury. Measures designed to save life, such as nursing in special or intensive care units, must have first priority but, as far as possible, arrangements are made for the parents to visit the unit frequently, to see, touch and handle their baby. Good communication between hospital and community nursing staff enables the midwife and health visitor to be aware of the need for additional support. Together with the medical social worker they give valuable counselling, which helps the parents through any difficulties so that possible effects of initial separation are overcome. This may be especially the case when a very small premature baby has remained in hospital for some time after the mother has returned home. Arrangements for visiting and feeding the baby, care of other children in the family and understanding support from the community midwife and health visitor can result in preservation of the bond in spite of initial difficulties.

Breast-feeding. The benefits of breast-feeding are well recognised from the aspect of protection against infection and reduction of the risk of allergy, as well as providing one of the best ways of establishing early communication between mother and child. Preparation for breast-feeding begins in the ante-natal months. Its establishment in the early neonatal period and successful continuation at home is of prime importance to health in the early years of life. The maintenance of successful breast-feeding, particularly in the first month, depends considerably on the understanding and consistent advice and practical assistance from the midwife and health visitor (Chapter 8).

Improvement of perinatal mortality

1 Health education before and during pregnancy
2 Early and regular attendance for ante-natal care; high standards of ante-natal care, including screening tests
3 Hospital delivery
4 Care at and following birth

The post-perinatal period

Out of every 1000 babies born alive, 994 enter the post-perinatal period (between the ages of one week and one year) and 988 of these will be alive at the end of their first year.

Concern is focused on the health of these infants, on the extent to which illness (morbidity) occurs and the reasons why a small group of children die. As in the perinatal period, there is a well-defined post-perinatal mortality rate. Morbidity can be expressed in terms of handicap and serious illness requiring notification of infection or admission to hospital. Surveys showing the reasons for consultation with the general practitioner may give some idea of the incidence of other conditions. There is virtually no statistical evidence on the frequency of minor symptoms which have not hitherto been recognised by parents or professional staff as having any potentially dangerous significance, although recent studies on infant deaths have accumulated limited data.

Post-perinatal mortality

Post-perinatal mortality is expressed as the number of children in any one year who die between the age of one week and one year per 1000 live births. Like the perinatal mortality rate, the post-perinatal mortality rate in this country has been declining, although the improvement in the last 20 years has been less marked than for the perinatal period, and figures remain higher than those of comparable countries (Table 3.1).

Causes of death   Possible ways of reducing the post-perinatal mortality rate may be indicated by an analysis of the causes of death in this period.

A few infants manage to survive the first seven days of life only to die in the second, third or fourth weeks from conditions similar to those associated with perinatal death, particularly low birth weight. These

Table 3.1 Mortality rates (1960–80) in England and Wales (see pages 51, 53, 58)

Year	Early neonatal	Perinatal	Post-perinatal	Infant
1960	13.3	32.8	8.5	21.8
1970	10.6	23.5	7.6	18.2
1975	9.1	19.3	6.7	15.7
1976	8.1	17.7	6.1	14.3
1977	7.6	17.0	6.1	13.8
1978	7.1	15.5	6.1	13.2
1979	6.8	14.7	6.1	12.8
1980	6.2	13.3	5.9	12.0

Source: Mortality statistics: childhood and maternity 1979, Series DH3 no.6 (HMSO 1981). Mortality statistics: childhood 1980, Series DH3 no.8 (HMSO 1982). Birth statistics 1980, Series FM1 no.7 (HMSO 1982).

numbers are comparatively small and, in general, deaths after the first week show a pattern of causes which is very different from that of the perinatal death. Fig. 3.4 shows a breakdown of deaths by cause.

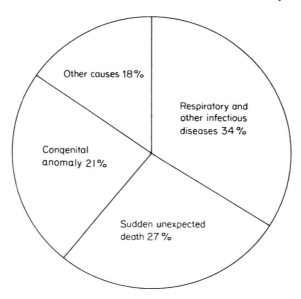

Fig. 3.4 Post-perinatal death by cause (1980)

In looking at the main causes of death from the aspect of prevention, main problem areas can be identified, with very different approaches to solutions:

Deaths due to abnormality.   Many major congenital defects such as those affecting the central nervous system, the renal system and the heart are by their very nature, once established, incompatible with long-continued life, although advances in surgery have greatly changed the outlook in some instances. To a great extent, death from these causes can be regarded as almost inevitable.

Deaths due to infection and 'sudden unexpected death'.   In some respects there would appear to be little reason for grouping these two categories of death together. In cases of severe infection, the child is clinically ill with recognisable symptoms and, in theory at least, the problem is relatively well defined. Sudden unexpected death, on the other hand, presents a complex and not fully understood problem. Children who are apparently well, in that they are not considered to need medical treatment, die at home unexpectedly—a devastating happening in itself for the family, and carrying with it a distressing aftermath of official enquiry, bewilderment, recrimination and frustration in the face of its inexplicability. In recent years, a great deal of research has been carried out in an attempt to explain this tragic happening. Certain features have emerged, notably the fact that the immediate cause of death is not necessarily the same for each child. Various theories have been put forward, such as disturbance of the normal reflex breathing responses (perhaps due to minimal brain damage at birth) and extreme allergic responses, but few as yet reveal a tangible, precise mechanism which could be altered so as to prevent death. Post-mortem findings may show minor degrees of infection, not severe enough ordinarily to cause death; in other instances there is evidence that the normal processes of growth have been retarded; in yet others, there are no abnormal findings whatsoever, death having occurred in a child who is apparently completely healthy.

One common link between deaths from acute infection and sudden unexpected death, is that on looking deeper into the total circumstances preceding death there often emerges the feeling that these are *not* deaths which should be considered as inevitable. Acute infections such as broncho-pneumonia, severe gastro-enteritis and meningitis do have a recognised mortality rate. There have been, however, such major advances in prevention, diagnosis and treatment (immunisation, modi-fied milk feeds, biochemical and bacteriological tests, and antibiotics) that the underlying factor in death seems to be related to the failure to make adequate use of preventive measures, and the failure to diagnose an illness and refer the child early enough for treatment to be effective. Many of these children die at home, even though hospital paediatric facilities are available, or arrive at hospital in a moribund condition. Their death would seem not to have been anticipated, and in this con-text they may be regarded as one end of the spectrum of unexpected death.

At the other end, where the more typical sudden (cot) deaths are concerned, recent studies have shown that here, too, death is not always as unexpected as it might at first appear. Detailed enquiries into the medical history preceding death and the social history of the child and family often reveal factors which add up to an unsatisfactory picture. These include minor symptoms of illness, changes in the usual pattern of the child's behaviour and responses such as unusual drowsiness, failure to maintain the expected rate of weight gain, low norms of health (which allow more major symptoms to be accepted without undue concern) and family stress. Despite these warning signs, the family, or indeed at times the professional health workers, do not always recognise that all is not well.

Reduction of post-perinatal mortality

Long-term reduction in post-perinatal mortality will depend on methods of preventing serious congenital defects and more effective methods of treatment for some viral infections. Much more research is also needed into the incidence of minor illness in children and the significance of common symptoms such as snuffles, coughs, and irritability, which may be pointers to some more serious underlying disturbance of health.

In the short-term, however, early diagnosis of illness, particularly severe acute infection and its prompt treatment, should produce more immediate reduction in post-perinatal deaths. The problem here appears to lie not so much in lack of facilities for treatment as in why help is not sought earlier. Where 'cot deaths' are concerned, although the exact mechanism of death may not be known and it may not, in every instance, be possible to identify at an early stage all the contributory factors, the answer may well hinge on adjusting some aspects of the total environment of the child and family. This would include a consideration of:

1 Community health services The majority of parents cope satisfactorily with the system for obtaining medical advice in the care of their child, but in a minority of instances, sometimes those where the need is most urgent, there is difficulty in obtaining help with disastrous consequences. The problem may lie in a variety of circumstances, for example:

(a) Lack of knowledge on the part of the parent as to what services there are and how to obtain them, particularly in unsocial hours.
(b) Difficulty of parents in communicating their need to the health worker concerned, particularly in the case of non-English speaking people.

(c)   Physical barriers such as vandalised telephones, and inconveniently sited clinics and surgeries.
(d)   Previous unfortunate experience with the health services leading to reluctance to consult again.

Prevention of post-perinatal deaths includes a critical examination of the ways in which community child health services are operating, so as to ensure that they are in practice, as well as in theory, appropriate, adequate, available and used to best advantage.

2   Child and family   Much work has been done to try to identify at an early age those children at increased risk of dying unexpectedly. Compilation of risk factors varies from complex statistical systems to the subjective opinions of health workers. Whatever the system, the babies who appear to be the most vulnerable are those born prematurely, twins, or the first baby of a very young mother. There is accumulating evidence that increased frequency of health visiting in the early months of life is saving the lives of some babies, particularly those considered to be at increased risk. It is difficult to single out any one specific aspect of health visitor activity which is helping to bring about this improvement. It is probably a summation of many factors:

(a)   The establishment of a sustained confident relationship with the mother.
(b)   Helping parents to know their child and to interpret the ways in which the baby attempts to communicate with them.
(c)   Education in the recognition of less obvious distress signals from the child and early signs of illness, and in the appropriate use of services.
(d)   Practical aspects of care, such as advice about feeding, and the monitoring of growth.

3   Co-ordination and communication   Many workers may be involved in the health care of the mother and young child—midwife, health visitor, general practitioner, clinic doctor, hospital paediatrician and social worker. Whilst each has his or her own expert contribution to make, it is important to ensure that knowledge about a child and family is shared, so as to build up the complete picture. After a death has occurred, it is often realised with hindsight that individual workers may each have held a piece of the puzzle, which if put together earlier might have altered the child's outcome. Time often precludes frequent interdisciplinary consultation, but thought could be given to the introduction of a child health record, held by the parent, and available for entries to be made and read by the medical and nursing staff caring for the family.

Prevention of post-perinatal mortality

1 Planning and use of community health services
2 Increased health visitor involvement with parent and child
3 Improved co-ordination and communication
4 Research into illness

Later mortality

After the first year, death in children is comparatively rare and the pattern of causes of death has changed (Table 3.2).

Table 3.2 Child mortality (1981)

	Ages 1–4 years	*Ages 5–14 years*
Rate	50 per 100 000 *total* population	24 per 100 000 *total* population
Commonest causes of death	1 Accident 2 Congenital abnormality 3 Respiratory	1 Accident 2 Malignancy 3 Congenital abnormality

Accidents in childhood

One aspect of the child/environment relationship, that of accidents, assumes alarming proportions in children over the age of one year. Accidents account for:

1 Over a quarter of all deaths in children aged 1–15.
2 One in five of all hospital admissions of children over the age of one.
3 One in six children attending accident and emergency departments.
4 Numbers of children becoming seriously and permanently handicapped.

The main areas where accidents occur are:

1 The road The highest proportion of accidents to children occurs on the road, particularly pedestrian accidents which tend to occur at times of excitement, such as coming out of school, or seeing a familiar figure across the road.

2   The home   Accidents of many kinds occur in the home, paradoxi-
cally the place where a child is considered safest. The more common
types of home accidents are:

(a)   *Injury* such as fractures and cuts caused by structural features.
      Modern house design often includes extensive use of glass in doors
      and picture windows, open staircases and balconies, all of which
      carry potential hazards for young children. At the other extreme,
      accidents are a hazard for children living in poor housing
      conditions with overcrowding.
(b)   *Poisoning* from the ingestion of medicines and tablets (often
      tantalisingly resembling sweets), household cleansing materials
      such as bleach and disinfectants, and gardening solutions such as
      weedkillers. In addition, an astounding variety of foreign bodies
      may be swallowed, from nails and coins to unlikely objects such as
      magnets.
(c)   *Burns and scalds* from the unguarded fire, play with matches,
      pulling over of pans and teapots, and handling of boiling liquids.

3   At play   Accidents here take on a variety of forms, such as those
occurring on playgrounds with poorly designed equipment, from the
hazards of popular crazes such as skateboards, or bathing accidents and
the ingestion of poisonous berries.

Prevention of accidents

The prevention of accidents in childhood is one of the big tasks of
preventive health, and depends upon a number of different approaches.

Education of parent and child   The majority of parents look on
protection of their child as one of the main obligations of parenthood
and are assiduous in their efforts to prevent harm occurring. It is,
however, virtually impossible to foresee every eventuality, and accidents
can occur in the split-second unguarded moment which occurs in the life
of every family. Nevertheless, there are some areas in which safety
education may be worthwhile:

1   Parents can be helped to understand the age at which a child may be
    expected to be aware of potential danger, and able to take steps for
    his own protection. Where road safety is concerned, it is particularly
    important for the parents to have a realistic appreciation of their
    child's capacity to take care of himself on a busy road and to
    understand and remember instructions. Motorists also should be
    aware of the unpredictable nature of a child's behaviour, so that
    caution can be exercised when approaching children or places where
    they congregate, such as schools and playgrounds. Steps are being

considered to include information on children's behaviour in the Highway Code. The Law forbids children riding in the front seat of a car unless a restraint is used. Evidence shows that there is also a risk of child back-seat passengers being seriously injured in car accidents and parents should be encouraged to provide restraints, even though there is at present no legal requirement.

2   The health visitor regards home safety as one of her priorities when she visits the home of a young child. She will notice points of possible danger and suggest ways by which the risk may be reduced, often being able to enlist the aid of other agencies such as the housing department and the environmental health department in remedying defects. It has been shown that stress in a family may increase considerably the risk of an accident involving the child and, in such a situation, the health visitor may be the key person to recognise and help alleviate the strain.

3   The importance of adult example should be stressed, particularly where road safety is concerned. Safety codes will only become meaningful to a child when other people are seen to be observing them also.

4   Organised campaigns directed towards special aspects of safety, such as the removal of unwanted drugs, are valuable in focusing attention on hazards, particularly if followed by a long-term programme of education (Fig. 3.5).

A safe environment   Potential danger in the environment, whether on the road, at home or at play is a factor with which both child and parents have to eventually come to terms. On the one hand, children have a natural curiosity and love of exploration and adventure through which they learn about the outside world, and which are to be encouraged if development is to take place. On the other hand, thought has to be given to ways in which the environment can be made reasonably accident-proof. To some extent this has already been achieved in the production of non-inflammable material for children's clothes, the fitting of compulsory guards to gas and electric fires, and the manufacture of child-proof containers for medicines. The latter are available on request to the chemist supplying the prescribed treatment, and parents may need to be made aware of this provision. More attention should also be given to improved house design and safe playground equipment.

Special provision   Many groups are involved in the prevention of accidents both at national and local level:

1   The Child Accident Prevention Committee is a national multi-disciplinary committee concerned with the prevention of all kinds of

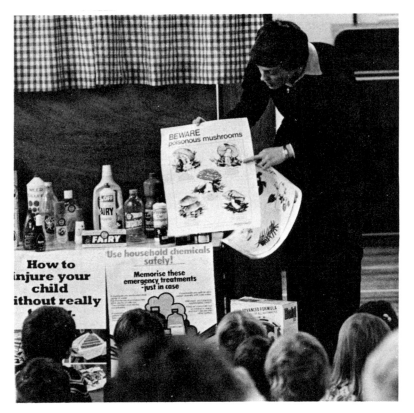

Fig. 3.5 Prevention of accidents—health education. *Colin New*

accidents to children and acts as a co-ordinating body for accident prevention.

2   Local home safety committees are usually set up by the environmental health departments of the local authority.

3   The Royal Society for the Prevention of Accidents (RoSPA) is a voluntary organisation which issues health education material on accident prevention, organises conferences and acts as a pressure group to encourage safer environmental conditions.

4   The home accident surveillance system is organised by the Department of Prices and Consumer Protection, and gives analyses of home accidents which are useful in pin-pointing the most urgent areas of concern.

5   Poison advice centres are set up in different parts of the country to give quick information on the effects of poison and the appropriate treatment.

Accidents in childhood

1 Occur at home, on the road, and at play
2 Prevention includes:
    health education for parent and child
    help from the health visitor
    adult example
    a safer environment
3 National and local organisations are involved in prevention

---

Malignant disease in childhood

Malignant disease in children, although the second commonest cause of death in the combined age group 1–15 years, is comparatively rare. It is estimated that approximately 1200 new cases are diagnosed in England and Wales each year, the most common form being acute lymphatic leukaemia. Big strides have been made in recent years in the treatment of childhood malignancy, and the prognosis is now greatly improved, more than 50 % surviving for over three years. Treatment usually involves a complicated regime of drug therapy, sometimes combined with surgery and radiotherapy, and is ideally undertaken in special regional oncology centres. A team which includes a paediatrician, surgeon, radiotherapist, nursing staff, medical social worker and laboratory staff is concerned not only with diagnosis and treatment, but also with helping to counsel and support the whole family, to whom the nature of the illness and, at times, the complications of therapy present distressing problems. As treatment continues, the child is usually able to spend varying periods of time at home, and the team co-ordinator (usually a consultant paediatrician), whilst maintaining overall supervision, links up closely with community medical and nursing staff, and social and educational services, to ensure that child and family receive the support and services they need (Chapter 9).

Reduction of later mortality

Although the death rate in children after the first year of life is small, it is hoped that future years will show a continuing fall. The two very different principal causes of death need different approaches to prevention. Reduction of deaths due to accident calls for an increased awareness, thought and action on the part of individuals and the community. The solution to the problem of malignancy is likely to be found within the more specialised field of research. It is hoped that measures to prevent death will also be efficacious in reducing handicap resulting from non-fatal accidents and in simplifying the treatment of malignant conditions.

Reduction of later mortality

1 Public and individual preventive action against accidents
2 Research into the causes and treatment of malignancy

4

Surveillance of Health I

Growth in the Early Years

Childhood is a time when the foundations for future health are laid down. A function of the community child health service is to arrange programmes of surveillance through which progress in all areas of a child's health can be observed and measured. This confirms normality in the majority of children and, in the few instances where departures from the expected pattern are detected, further investigation can be arranged. Many different professional staff participate in surveillance; the basic programme is usually undertaken by a doctor, health visitor or school nurse, but sometimes includes the teacher, educational psychologist, orthoptist, speech therapist or audiometrician. Surveillance procedures can be carried out in the home, a well-child clinic, day nursery or school.

Surveillance offers a splendid opportunity for the child's progress to be discussed by professional workers and parents together, and explanation of the procedures helps parents to understand the pattern and sequence of growth and development. Surveillance includes the history of the child, his family and social background, and a series of observations, examinations and tests appropriate to the child's age.

The history

The history enables any findings that emerge as a result of surveillance procedures to be considered not only in the context of the whole child, but also of his family circumstances and relationships and of the community in which they live. Relevant points to be discussed are:

1 The family's medical history, which might indicate inherited tendencies or abnormal conditions which could affect the child's growth and development.
2 Events in the pre-natal and perinatal periods which may have some significance for future progress e.g. prematurity.
3 Progress since birth. The first examination is usually carried out shortly after birth in the hospital neonatal unit and serves as a baseline for future screening.
4 The social and cultural background of the family, which includes:

   (a) The parents' occupations, the size of the family, the degree of affluence or poverty, and housing conditions.

(b) Special circumstances such as the one-parent family, the ethnic origin of the family (particularly in relation to cultural customs and practices) and the understanding of the English language.
5 The parents' own observations on their child's progress and behaviour, and any episode of stress or change in the family circumstances.
6 Where relevant, the reports of the teacher on the educational progress of a child of school age.

Information about a child includes:

1 Family history
2 Pre-natal and perinatal circumstances
3 Post-natal progress
4 The social and cultural background of the family
5 The parents' observations
6 Where relevant, the teacher's comments

Surveillance will be discussed under four broad headings:

1 Observation of growth (Chapter 4)
2 Physical examination (Chapter 5)
3 Developmental screening (Chapter 6)
4 Health and education (Chapter 7)

Observation of growth

Growth is a sign of life and health. Each individual child shows varying rhythms of growth which change throughout infancy and childhood. Growth is influenced by many interacting factors, some of which are to be found within the child himself, some in his environment.

Factors within the child

Heredity The general control of growth is determined by the action of many genes which together influence the rate of growth, the time when it will cease and the potential height which an individual can reach. These genes are helped to achieve their full effect by good environmental conditions.

The endocrine system Several endocrine organs produce hormones which influence growth. The pituitary gland plays an important part by producing a specific growth hormone and controls the function of other glands, such as the thyroid and adrenals.

Illness   Acute or chronic illness or congenital abnormality may lead to disturbance of growth.

Factors in the environment

Diet   Certain nutritional factors are needed to promote growth, maintain the body systems and repair wear and tear. A balanced diet includes various foods which together supply all the essential nutrients. The most important constituents in the diet are:

1   Proteins containing essential amino-acids. Protein is necessary for growth and tissue repair and is valuable in enabling the pituitary gland to fulfil its growth functions adequately.
2   Minerals such as sodium, iron and calcium, which have specific functions—for example, sodium helps to maintain the chemical balance of the body, iron is needed for haemoglobin production, and calcium is essential for bone and teeth formation.
3   Vitamins, which are complex chemical compounds, and are necessary in small amounts to maintain bodily functions. Vitamin D encourages the growth of bone and teeth, Vitamin C maintains the health of connective tissue and contributes to resistance to infection, and the B vitamins aid the function of many parts of the body, particularly the nervous system.
4   Fats and carbohydrates supplying most of the energy requirements of the body.

Emotional factors   Good parental care includes the provision of a loving, secure environment for the child and it has been suggested that this helps in the production of pituitary growth hormones (Fig. 4.1).

Growth is encouraged by:

1   Genetic factors
2   Adequate endocrine function
3   Freedom from illness
4   Good nutrition
5   Secure loving home

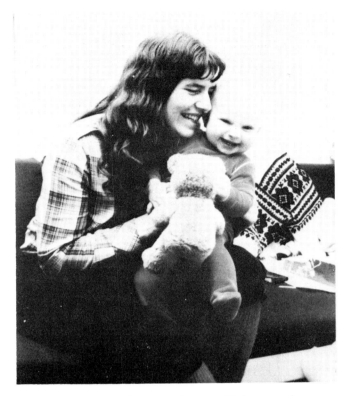

Fig. 4.1   A loving environment helps growth

Measurement of growth

For practical general purposes, three measurements of growth are commonly made:

1 *Weight.* The birthweight of a baby gives a base-line from which to record, at intervals, weight changes throughout the child's life.
2 *Height (or length).* This is not easy to measure accurately in a small baby, and is a more appropriate measurement for the older infant or child who can stand erect and remain relatively still for a short time.
3 *Head circumference.* Measurement of the head circumference is extremely important during the first two years of life, particularly so in the first six months. The head is measured by passing a clearly marked narrow non-stretchable tape measure firmly round the head just above the base of the nose and over the occipital prominence.

> *Measurements of growth*
> 1 Weight
> 2 Height after first year
> 3 Head circumference in the first two years

Single measurements, whether of weight, height or head circumference, observed in isolation have very limited value. Much more helpful are serial measurements, by means of which a present reading can be compared with preceding ones. A percentile chart gives a clear, easily understood picture of the rate of growth and enables unexpected variations to be detected early (Fig. 4.2).

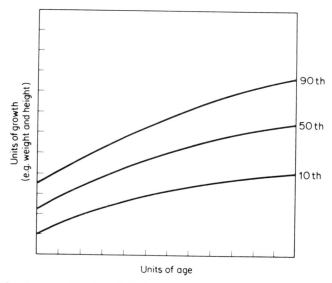

Fig. 4.2 A percentile chart in infant growth (diagrammatic). A line labelled 10th percentile indicates that for any given unit of age, in large numbers of children, 10 % would have weights below the line, 90 % above

Each child has his own individual growth pattern. In normal growth, the measurements usually follow a steady path relative to any one percentile line—for example, weight, starting on the 50th percentile at birth, tends to remain on this line at succeeding ages. In addition, each measurement, whether of weight, height or head circumference, should lie on the corresponding percentile line—for example, a child whose weight lies on the 10th percentile line would also have height and head circumference on the corresponding 10th line. Continued divergence from one percentile line towards another, or disproportion as shown by weight/ height or weight/head circumference being on different percentile lines, may indicate abnormality and need investigation.

Variations of growth causing concern

In the majority of children, growth as a whole proceeds steadily and uneventfully. In some children, however, disturbances of growth arise which need investigation. The following will be considered:

1 Failure to thrive
2 Obesity
3 Short stature
4 Abnormal rates of growth of the head circumference

Failure to thrive

The use of percentile charts gives early warning of failure to thrive before the more obvious signs of weight standstill or loss become evident (Fig. 4.3).

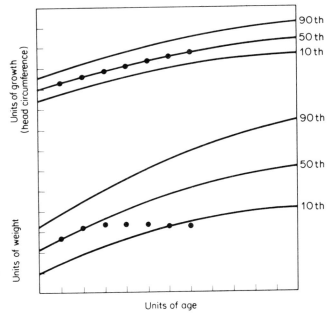

Fig. 4.3   A percentile chart in failure to thrive (diagrammatic)

Because the health visitor or school nurse is frequently involved in weighing children, she is often the first person to become aware that a child is not thriving, and may be able to uncover contributory factors. Time spent in discussion with the parents is very rewarding, and a home visit presents the opportunity to assess the domestic circumstances and observe the relationship between mother and child.

The reason for failure to thrive may be primarily within the child, but is more commonly due to environmental factors.

Environmental factors

Inadequate intake of food The diet may be inadequate in quantity or quality, or both. It is helpful to discuss the diet in some detail, to visit at a meal-time, obtain information about the food taken in the past 24 hours, observe breast-feeding and, in the case of a bottle-fed baby, to watch the mother make-up a feed and give it to the child. A variety of factors may come to light:

1 Ignorance about the elementary principles of nutrition.
2 Inability to read or understand instructions.
3 Difficulties in maintaining breast-feeding, or mechanical difficulties in bottle-feeding, such as too small a hole in the teat.
4 A diet restricted by cultural and religious patterns.
5 A family income insufficient to provide enough food of the right kind.

The health visitor may need to increase the frequency of her visits to the family. She will provide education on diet, using a variety of teaching methods and will advise on available financial benefits.

Psycho-social factors

Failure to thrive may stem primarily from disturbed relationships within the home. Inadequate provision of food may be the result of wilful neglect on the part of parents or of psychiatric disturbance, such as depression in parents, particularly the mother. The child himself may react to stress by a diminished appetite in spite of sufficient food being available. Another child eats food apparently adequate in quantity and quality but the emotional disturbance within himself is sufficient to affect his ability to utilise what he eats. The marked feature of all these children is their response of improved growth to removal to an environment of caring concern and adequate diet, which enables them to function in a more normal way. Their long-term management includes much patient work with the parents to help them provide a home environment and a loving relationship in which growth can proceed.

Factors within the child

Illness or abnormality Congenital heart disease, mental retardation and chronic infections may result in failure to thrive; the vomiting associated with pyloric stenosis leads to continued loss of nutrients. Chronic diarrhoea may have a similar effect. Local disorders such as severe thrush or cleft palate may cause feeding difficulties.

Inadequate utilisation of food Failure to thrive may be due to an inability to absorb or metabolise some essential nutrients of the diet owing to conditions such as cystic fibrosis, coeliac disease, lactose and milk protein intolerance, and diabetes.

Cystic fibrosis This is an inherited condition in which the glandular secretions of different organs throughout the body are altered. The pancreas fails to produce sufficient digestive enzymes to ensure the complete digestion and absorption of protein and fat, and nutrition may be seriously impaired. The tracheal secretions become abnormally thick leading to recurrent respiratory infection. A combination of failure to thrive in spite of a hearty appetite, the passage of bulky, pale, offensive, fatty stools, and a chronic cough should arouse a suspicion of cystic fibrosis. The clinical diagnosis can be confirmed by examining the sweat for increased salt content or by a special blood test.

Treatment:

1   Pancreatic enzymes are added to the diet in the form of granules, powder or capsules. The amount of fat in the diet is restricted to what is found to be tolerated, and special easily digestible fat supplements are available. Extra vitamins are also given.

2   Prevention of respiratory infection is important. This entails avoidance of crowded places and obvious sources of infection in the child's immediate circle. Immunisation is actively encouraged. Advice regarding smoking, both in the family and the older patient, is even more urgent than in ordinary circumstances. Regular physiotherapy is needed and this can be carried out by the parents after instruction from the physiotherapist. For some children antibiotics are prescribed on a regular basis or, in other instances, are reserved for an acute infection.

There is evidence to suggest that early active treatment, whilst not curing the condition, considerably reduces the severity of the symptoms and improves the expectation of life. The parents are given explanation of the condition, the treatment and services available and are helped to recognise the importance of their participation in treatment. Co-ordination of hospital and community services enables maximum help to be given (Chapter 9), and the Cystic Fibrosis Society offers information leaflets and support groups for parents. Early diagnosis also enables the parents to receive genetic counselling before considering another pregnancy, as the risk of a future child being similarly affected is 1 in 4. The incidence of cystic fibrosis is 1 in 1800 live births. Screening includes tests on the sweat, meconium, faeces and blood.

Coeliac disease Coeliac disease arises from an intolerance to gluten, the protein part of many cereals including wheat, rye and barley, and results in damage to the lining of the small intestine with consequent inadequate absorption of food. It occurs in 1 in 2000 people and may start at any time after the first 4–6 months of life, the stage at which gluten is commonly introduced into the weaning diet of babies. It is thought that later weaning (i.e. at six months) on a diet based on rice (which is gluten-free) rather than wheat cereals may prevent the development of gluten intolerance. The classical signs of coeliac disease are:

1 A thin, miserable child with a poor appetite, failing to thrive.
2 A protuberant abdomen.
3 Loss of superficial fat, particularly over the buttocks and thighs.
4 Anaemia.
5 Stools which, like those of cystic fibrosis, are very bulky, pale, frothy and highly offensive.

The diagnosis of coeliac disease is confirmed by jejunal biopsy. Histological examination of the jejunal mucosa shows a characteristic flattening of the villi which are normally deeply indented.

Treatment: Coeliac disease can be treated successfully by a high protein gluten-free diet. Children start to put on weight once gluten has been excluded from the diet and it is now thought that the gluten-free diet should be continued indefinitely, particularly from the aspect of prevention of growth retardation. Hospital and community dietitians and the health visitor work closely together to explain to parents the importance of the diet, and advise as to how gluten-free food or flour can be obtained; the Coeliac Society issues regularly a list of gluten-free products. Arrangements for suitable meals for the school-child can be made through the school health service and the school meals supervisior.

Lactose intolerance A small proportion of babies are unable to utilise lactose in milk; this may be congenital in origin, but more commonly develops as a temporary feature following gastro-enteritis, particularly in babies under the age of six months. They develop signs of failure to thrive and a watery diarrhoea causing excoriated buttocks; the fluid part of the stools contains sugar. A lactose-free substitute milk should be used.

Milk protein intolerance   Persistent diarrhoea and failure to thrive may be due to an intolerance to the protein in cows' milk, which may be triggered off by an episode of acute gastro-enteritis. Treatment is by giving a substitute milk containing soya protein or hydrolysed casein.

Diabetes   Diabetes results from an inability of the pancreas to produce sufficient insulin for the metabolism of sugar. One of the symptoms may be failure to thrive. Diabetes is discussed in more detail in Chapter 9.

When the reason for failure to thrive does not become apparent or cannot satisfactorily be dealt with in the home, hospital referral may be indicated. Many paediatric units provide day facilities for observation and education on nutrition. Children with suspected pathological conditions or psycho-social growth failure may need in-patient investigation and treatment.

Causes of failure to thrive

1   Food intake is inadequate
2   Psycho-social factors
3   General or local illness or abnormality
4   Inadequate utilisation of food:
     Cystic fibrosis
     Coeliac disease
     Lactose intolerance
     Milk protein intolerance
     Diabetes

Obesity

At the opposite end of the scale from failure to thrive is the problem of obesity. Fat babies show an increased susceptibility to respiratory infection and may be delayed in learning to walk. They do not always become fat children, but when obesity does occur in childhood it tends to persist into adolescence and adulthood. Prevention of childhood obesity can be an investment for future health in terms of reducing the risk of later diabetes, hypertension and ischaemic heart disease. Many interacting factors may result in obesity.

Factors within the child

Genetic factors If one or both parents are overweight, there is an increased chance that their child will be also. A genetic predisposition to obesity may be aggravated by family eating habits.

Endocrine factors Obesity may form part of specific syndromes due to endocrine disturbances, but these are comparatively rare causes.

Factors in the environment

Dietary intake and energy output The basic factor in obesity is frequently that the calorie intake in the diet is in excess of the energy expenditure of the body, and so fat is laid down. This is a very individual issue—some children gain more weight than others on precisely the same (or even less) calorie intake, and this may be accounted for by the differing degrees of energy expenditure.

Emotional factors Food, particularly that of high carbohydrate content, may act as a source of comfort for children where relationships in the home are strained or disturbed. A vicious circle develops— insecurity leads to overeating and to obesity which, in turn, produces social isolation or criticism for which solace is sought in increased eating.

Management of obesity

It is much easier to prevent obesity than to treat it, once it is firmly established. The regular recording of weight on a percentile chart (Fig. 4.4) will indicate when the rate of weight gain is becoming excessive and enable adjustments to dietary intake, such as reduction in carbo-hydrates, to be made. Breast-fed babies are less likely to become over-weight than bottle-fed babies and health education during the ante-natal period directed towards the encouragement of breast-feeding is a good preventive measure. The present trend to wait until the baby is six months of age before solids are introduced into the diet also reduces the risk of obesity.

Factors underlying obesity

1 Genetic predisposition
2 Endocrine disorders
3 Energy intake in diet exceeds energy output
4 Emotional factors

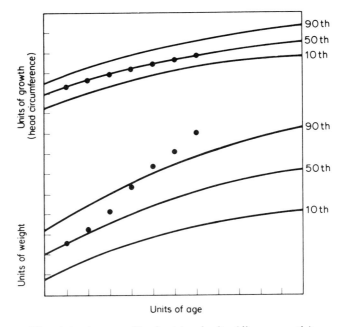

Fig. 4.4 A percentile chart in obesity (diagrammatic)

Short stature

Concern about short stature should arise when the height of a child is below the third centile or is only increasing very slowly (Fig. 4.5). The parents and the child himself may express anxiety arising out of comparison with other children of more average height. The causes of short stature arise from factors very similar to those which influence overall growth. Early recognition and identification of the cause are important as, in some instances, treatment can be successful in preventing permanent stunting of stature. The aim should be to identify unusually short stature before the age of seven, and preferably sooner.

Factors in the child

Heredity   There is often a family history of short stature—short parents are likely to have a short child. A particular chromosome abnormality involving the sex chromosome shows in 1 in 3000 girls as Turner's syndrome, one characteristic of which is short stature. This condition can be confirmed by chromosome analysis.

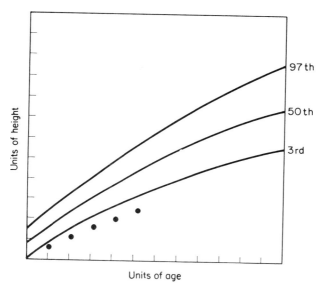

Fig. 4.5 A percentile chart in short stature (diagrammatic)

Specific growth hormone deficiency Failure of the pituitary gland to produce adequate amounts of growth hormone is the cause of short stature in a small proportion of children (1 in 10 000). This condition can be diagnosed by specific tests and responds to replacement treatment with growth hormone, the best results being obtained when it is started early, preferably by the age of 5–7 years.

Illness Some chronic conditions such as severe asthma, pyelonephritis, undiagnosed coeliac disease and hypothyroidism can cause slowing of growth. In addition, treatment which involves the use of steroids calls for a fine judgement in achieving the balance between the therapeutic dose and one which could cause secondary stunting of stature.

Environmental factors

Overall genetic control of height may be encouraged and modified by factors in the child's environment. A good environment helps in the attainment of the maximum height allowed by genetic make-up and, conversely, the full height may not be achieved if adverse environmental factors persist.

Good nutrition, both before and after birth, plays an important part in relation to increase in height. Poor social conditions associated with large family size, low income and inadequate diet can lead to slowing of growth and stunting of stature. Identification of socially deprived families may enable some degree of immediate help to be given in terms of any financial support to which they are entitled, free milk and school meals (Chapter 1).

Psycho-social factors may cause lack of growth in height as part of the general picture of failure to thrive.

Factors underlying short stature

1 Genetic causes
2 Growth hormone deficiency
3 Chronic illness or its treatment
4 Poor nutrition
5 Psycho-social factors

Variations in head circumference

Serial measurements of head circumference plotted on a percentile chart and noted in conjunction with weight recordings will give early warning of too-rapid or too-slow rate of increase in size (Fig. 4.6).

Too rapid rate of growth   The most common cause is *hydrocephalus*, an increase in the amount of cerebro-spinal fluid in the brain which eventually will fail to grow normally because of the raised intra-cranial pressure.

A less common cause, though equally important to recognise in the early stages, is subdural haematoma, an accumulation of blood beneath the dura mater, the fibrous covering of the brain. In a young baby this is usually the result of deliberate injury to the child.

Early recognition that the head circumference is increasing in size too rapidly enables early diagnosis of the cause to be made and appropriate treatment started.

Too slow rate of growth   *Microcephalus* is a congenital abnormality in which the brain is under-developed and fails to grow normally, and is characterised by a small head circumference at birth which continues to be disproportionate to other measurements. There is no treatment to cure this condition and microcephalic children are always mentally retarded.

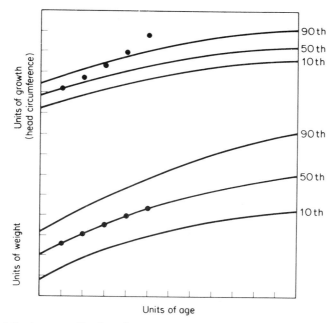

Fig. 4.6 A percentile chart in progressive hydrocephalus (diagrammatic)

The fontanelles

As well as measuring the head circumference, opportunity should be taken gently to feel the main fontanelles. The posterior fontanelle in the occipital region normally closes about the tenth day of life, but the larger anterior one remains palpable up to the age of eighteen months. Delayed closure may indicate hydrocephalus or rickets. The tension of the anterior fontanelle is important to feel—a tense, bulging fontanelle occurs in hydrocephalus and meningitis; a depressed fontanelle signifies severe dehydration. Observation should also be made of the shape of the head, noting any unusual degree of asymmetry or unusual contour.

A baby's head

1 Measure circumference
2 Feel fontanelles
3 Observe shape

The future

Today's children as a whole achieve much higher standards of growth, particularly in height, than those of preceding generations. This improvement is the result of advances on several fronts. Standards of living have improved and better nutrition, in particular, has played an important part. More is known of how growth is controlled, and the ways in which specific adverse factors can be identified and their effects treated. The increasing use of programmes of surveillance is helping to diagnose early those children with disturbed growth patterns, some of whom can be helped with appropriate treatment.

In the future, advances in medicine will undoubtedly result in more chronic illnesses being prevented, or their treatment refined so that their adverse effects on growth will be reduced. The development of more reliable screening tests will enable even earlier identification of potentially growth-limiting conditions. Improved ante-natal and perinatal care, both in the social and medical fields, should reduce the number of low birthweight babies. The huge problem that remains to be tackled concerns that of the conditions of social deprivation in which some children and their families are living, particularly in the inner-city areas. It is hoped that national and local policies will be co-ordinated so that housing will be improved and further financial support given, thereby reducing inequalities in health and enabling each child to achieve his full potential for growth.

5
Surveillance of Health II

Other Aspects of Physical Health in the Early Years

Monitoring of physical health is part of the total health surveillance of the child. In addition to the measurements of growth described in Chapter 4, methods of assessing physical health include:

1 Specific screening tests which identify some conditions whose successful treatment depends on early pre-symptomatic detection.
2 Physical examination of the child.

Specific screening tests

Screening tests are simple procedures which can be carried out on large numbers of children in order to detect, in a proportion of them, specific conditions for which treatment is available. Three scree ing tests are commonly carried out in the first week of a child's life:

1 The Ortolani test (or Barlow's modification) for congenital dislocation of the hip joint.
2 The Guthrie test to detect phenylketonuria.
3 Thyroid hormone assay to detect congenital hypothyroidism.

Congenital dislocation of the hip

This condition occurs when the head of the femur slips abnormally easily out of the acetabulum. To enable the joint to function normally, the femoral head must remain firmly in the acetabulum, so early diagnosis of instability and prompt treatment are important. It is estimated that one or two babies out of every 100 born in this country have unstable hips at birth.

Detection of instability or actual dislocation of the hip is possible by using Barlow's modification of the Ortolani test, which forms part of the neo-natal examination of a baby. This is based on gentle abduction of the thigh with the hip and knee in flexion and identification of the position and movement of the femoral head relative to the acetabulum. Even though the results of the test are satisfactory in the early days, the range of hip abduction should be checked again in the first few months.

This test can be done by a doctor, health visitor or midwife after appropriate training. A baby with a hip joint thought to be unstable is referred to an orthopaedic consultant who will decide on the appropriate treatment.

Treatment: Dislocation of the hip joint usually responds very well to early splinting, using a von Rosen or similar splint which is moulded to fit the individual baby and holds the head of the femur securely in the acetabulum. The splint is retained for two or three months, at least, and during that time must not be removed. The mother is reassured that the splint will not interfere with feeding (even breast-feeding), bathing or toileting.

Congenital dislocation of the hip

1 Early detection by Barlow test
2 Treatment by splinting

Phenylketonuria (PKU)

This condition arises as a result of the incomplete metabolism of phenylalanine, one of the essential amino-acids necessary for growth, which is found in normal protein diet. In a small number of children (approximately 1 in 6000) the liver fails to manufacture sufficient amounts of an enzyme needed for the complete breakdown of phenylalanine. This leads to an accumulation of toxic intermediate products which damage the developing brain cells of the child and cause mental retardation.

Detection of phenylketonuria at an early stage is most important as treatment can then be instituted which will enable growth and development to proceed normally. The Guthrie test detects high phenylalanine levels in the blood and should be carried out between day 6 and day 14 of life. Specimens of blood obtained from a heel-prick are transferred to a special absorbent filter paper and sent for biochemical examination. The blood is usually taken by the hospital or community midwife, or health visitor, depending on whether the baby is still in the hospital unit or at home at the relevant time. In some areas an alternative test (the Schriver test) analyses blood collected in a capillary tube. When a suspiciously high level of phenylalanine in the blood is found, further investigation is indicated to confirm or otherwise the diagnosis of phenylketonuria. Careful recording and cross-checking with birth notifications ensures that every baby is tested, the result noted and referral for further investigation arranged, if necessary. Very occasionally a parent may be unwilling for the Guthrie test to be done on the baby even though its importance is explained. In such a case it is advisable to test the baby's urine for phenylketones between the ages of 3–6 weeks, using a special strip paper (Phenistix). This test (known as the 'nappy test') is not as reliable as the Guthrie test, is not valid at a very early age and should only be used when a blood test is not practicable.

Treatment: Phenylketonuria usually responds well to a dietary regime in which enough essential nutrients for growth and development are provided, but the amounts of phenylalanine are strictly controlled, so as not to incur abnormally high blood levels. Regular blood tests are necessary to monitor the effectiveness of the diet, and are specially important when circumstances such as intercurrent infectious illness may temporarily upset the child's appetite.

The treatment and control of phenylketonuria involves many health staff. Paediatricians, biochemists and dietitians contribute to the diagnosis, establishment of treatment and monitoring of its effectiveness. Support and encouragement from general practitioners and health visitors are invaluable in helping parents to come to terms with the situation and understand the necessity for the child to adhere strictly to the diet. When school age is reached, special arrangements regarding school meals are made through the school health service and the school meals supervisor. There is no general rule as to how long the diet should be continued. Much depends on the response of the individual child, but it is thought at least until the early teens.

Successful treatment means that girls with phenylketonuria are reaching child-bearing age as normal healthy individuals, but special precautions are needed when pregnancy is contemplated. It is essential that the special diet is carefully continued or reintroduced prior to conception and maintained throughout pregnancy, with regular blood phenylalanine estimation. This helps to prevent abortion or fetal damage which could result from high phenylalanine levels in the mother's blood.

Phenylketonuria is a genetically determined condition and arises when a child inherits from each parent a recessive gene which prevents the enzyme formation in the liver. The risk that a subsequent child of the same parents will also have phenylketonuria is 1 in 4, and genetic counselling is advisable to help the parents appreciate the significance of a future pregnancy.

Phenylketonuria

1 An inherited abnormality of protein metabolism
2 Early detection by the Guthrie test
3 Treated by strict special diet
4 Extra precautions during pregnancy
5 Genetic counselling for parents and affected older girls

Congenital hypothyroidism

Hormones produced by the thyroid gland are essential for growth and development. Untreated congenital hormone deficiency, particularly of thyroxine, results in the condition of *cretinism*. Characteristic signs of hypothyroidism are:

1 *In the very young baby*: lethargy and lack of alertness, a large protruding tongue, a hoarse cry, umbilical hernia, slow feeding and constipation, sometimes prolonged jaundice, and failure to thrive.
2 *Going on to*: developmental delay, mental retardation and growth retardation.

It is estimated that one child in 2700–5000 suffers from under-activity of the thyroid gland at birth.

Hypothyroidism may be very difficult to detect by clinical examination immediately after birth, and the physical signs tend to develop only gradually over the first few weeks of life. It is now possible to screen young babies for hypothyroidism by carrying out a hormone analysis on blood taken at the same time as that for the Guthrie test (between day 6 and day 14).

Treatment of hypothyroidism by carefully regulated thyroxine replacement therapy promotes normal growth and development. The earlier the treatment is started, the more complete the response—particularly where mental development is concerned. Screening programmes for congenital hypothyroidism are still in their early days and will be evaluated through careful follow-up by clinical and biochemical examination of the progress of the children needing treatment.

Congenital hypothyroidism

1 A deficiency of thyroid hormones
2 Early detection is possible by estimation of thyroid hormone in the blood
3 Early treatment by thyroxine produces normal development

Physical examination

Physical examination of the child has for a long time been regarded as a traditional form of surveillance and parents, in particular, tend to feel that no health assessment is complete without it. It has been shown, however, that repeated physical examination does not necessarily add to our knowledge of a normal healthy child, and it is important to define the circumstances in which it will prove most valuable. Physical examination is indicated:

1 To identify congenital defects. Most of the major characteristics are found in the first neo-natal examination but a few, particularly congenital heart defects, may not show clinical signs until a few weeks later.
2 When the parents or teachers are worried about a child's health.
3 When assessment in other fields, such as growth and development, indicate a need—for example, failure to thrive or delay in walking.
4 When a previous examination has not been satisfactory, or there is any specific cause for anxiety such as suspicion of non-accidental injury.

Routine physical examinations over and above measurements of growth, specific screening tests and developmental screening are usually needed on two or three occasions only in the first five years of the child's life, and include examination of the main systems of the body.

The skeletal system

Examination establishes the normality of the limbs, head, spine and thorax, and excludes congenital defects such as instability of the hip joint and talipes. Some parents may express concern about what they consider to be an unusual gait or abnormal stance in their child. Conditions labelled by them as 'flat-feet', 'knock-knees' or 'bow-legs' are often nothing more than the normal variation of posture or appearance which change as walking and the acquisition of balance are achieved. In most cases explanation and reassurance are all that is needed. The experienced examiner will be able to distinguish physiological variation from conditions which, especially if accompanied by pain or a limp, require referral for an orthopaedic or paediatric opinion.

Rickets One cause of pronounced bowing of the legs and knock-knee is rickets,which is caused by Vitamin D deficiency. Vitamin D is essential in the absorption of calcium from the intestine for utilisation in the ossification of bone from cartilage. Deficiency of Vitamin D arises when lack of sunshine prevents its natural manufacture in the skin and the dietary intake is poor. It can occur in children of any ethnic group but is more likely in those of Asian origin, probably because of a combination of their dark skins, dietary habits and ignorance of the use of vitamin supplements. Rickets may occur:

1 In the neo-natal period in babies born to mothers whose diet has been severely deficient in Vitamin D or in the very small premature baby. This is often accompanied by twitching and tetany.
2 Between the ages of six months to three years. Important signs are general irritability and fretfulness, flabbiness of muscles which may lead to delay in walking, thickening of the wrists, softening of the skull bones with delayed closure of the anterior fontanelle and bowing of the tibia when weight-bearing on the legs begins. X-ray of the wrist shows a characteristic appearance of the lower end of the radius and ulna. Blood tests may show raised alkaline phosphatase levels before any other abnormality is present.
3 In adolescence, when pain in the legs is an early sympton. The pain, together with tiredness and muscle weakness becomes increasingly severe and disabling and, unless its significance is realised, serious deformities of the legs and pelvis occur.

Treatment: The aim of treatment is to remedy the underlying Vitamin D deficiency before irreversible bone changes occur. Oral preparation such as Adexolin are effective when early diagnosis is made. Severe cases may need, initially, a more concentrated form of Vitamin D. Improvement is maintained by a diet adequate in Vitamin D and the use of vitamin supplements.

Rickets is a preventable condition and success depends on:

1 The awareness of risk, particularly amongst people of Asian origin.
2 Health education regarding diet and the need for vitamin supplements.
3 Information on how vitamin supplements can be obtained.

Prevention presents a challenge to health education in non-English speaking communities. Information can be disseminated through pictorial leaflets and posters (Fig. 5.1), films with commentaries in the common Asian languages, and programmes on the media. Most important of all is the involvement of health visitors, school nurses, community nurses, teachers, dietitians, doctors, and social workers in health education on a personal or small group basis. Help should be enlisted from official interpreters, community relations officers, leaders of religious communities and volunteers who work in schemes for the teaching of English to Asian women.

Rickets

1 Caused by Vitamin D deficiency
2 More common in Asian children
3 Can be prevented
4 Early diagnosis to prevent deformity

آپ کے بچے کو وٹامن ڈی کی ضرورت ہے . . . . تاکہ اس کی ہڈیاں مضبوط رہیں ۔

Your child needs Vitamin D
. . . to keep his bones strong.

جس وقت آپ کے بچے کی جلد پر سورج کے شعاع میں پڑتی ہیں، اس کا بدن خود بخود وٹامن ڈی بنالیتا ہے ۔

When the *sun* shines on the child's skin, the body makes its own Vitamin D.

لیکن اس ملک میں سورج زیادہ نظر نہیں آتا ۔

But there is not much sun in this country.

چنانچہ آپ کے بچے میں وٹامن ڈی کی کمی ہوسکتی ہے۔ جس کی وجہ سے اس کی ہڈیاں ٹیڑھی ہوسکتی ہیں ۔

So your child could be short of Vitamin D. This could cause his bones to bend.

اس صورتِ حال سے بچنے کے لئے آپ دو کام کرسکتے ہیں ۔

You can do two things to prevent this happening . . . give him vitamin drops. These contain Vitamin D.

بچے کو وٹامن کے قطرے دیں۔ ان میں وٹامن ڈی شامل ہوتا ہے ۔

Give him, and all the family, foods that contain Vitamin D.

اس کو اور سب افرادِ خاندان کو ایسی غذا دیں جس میں وٹامن ڈی شامل ہو ۔

Butter is good, but margarine contains even more Vitamin D. *You can buy vegetarian margarine and make ghee with it.*

مکھن اچھی چیز ہے ۔ مگر مارجرین میں اس سے بھی زیادہ وٹامن ڈی ہوتا ہے ۔ آپ سبزی والا مارجرین خرید کر اس سے گھی بنا سکتے ہیں ۔

Eggs and oily fish, such as sardines, mackerel and herring, contain lots of Vitamin D.

انڈے اور تیل والی مچھلیاں مثلاً سارڈین، میکریل اور ہیرنگ میں وٹامن ڈی کثرت سے پایا جاتا ہے ۔

Your doctor or health visitor will tell you where to get the drops, and how much to give your child. Do not give more than you are told. Too much can be harmful.

آپ کے ڈاکٹر یا ہیلتھ وزیٹر یہ بتا سکتے ہیں کہ یہ قطرے کہاں سے حاصل کئے جا سکتے ہیں ۔ اور کتنی مقدار بچے کو دینی چاہئے۔ آپ کو جو ہدایت کی گئی ہو اس سے زیادہ نہ دیں۔ ضرورت سے زیادہ دینے سے بھی نقصان ہوسکتا ہے ۔

Fig. 5.1 Health education on rickets—Urdu and English

Ears and eyes

A great part of the examination of ears and eyes is concerned with their functional use in the development of hearing and vision, respectively, and will be discussed in Chapter 6. Early detection of congenital cataracts is important as prompt referral for specialist advice is indicated. Surgical treatment before the age of 8 weeks and subsequent fitting of special contact lenses greatly improve the chances of normal vision developing.

The heart and circulatory system

Some congenital heart defects are not always clinically apparent in the first few days of life and this forms a cogent reason for further examination at the age of six weeks. Any cyanosis or rapid breathing is observed. Auscultation of the heart may reveal a murmur. Many heart murmurs are functional in origin; they are of no serious import and discretion should be used as to whether or not mention should be made to the parents. An experienced doctor is usually able to distinguish between functional murmurs and those which indicate a cardiac defect and need further investigation. The femoral pulses are palpated to exclude coarctation of the aorta—a congenital narrowing of the descending aorta which can result in a lessened flow of blood through the femoral arteries. Failure to thrive may be a presenting sign in some cases of congential heart defect.

The respiratory system

The most common problems of the respiratory tract are those associated with infection. A single routine examination reveals the state of affairs on that particular occasion only and most examinations are carried out at the request of parents who are concerned about coughs, colds and chronic catarrh.

The abdomen

Palpation of the abdomen is usual in order to detect any enlargement of the liver and spleen. In the young baby palpation of the inguinal region may reveal an inguinal hernia for which early surgical treatment, usually on a day-patient or short-stay basis, is advised.

The genito-urinary system

Early routine examination should always include confirmation that the testes are descended.

Undescended testes In 97 % of full-term male babies, both testes are fully descended at birth and can be palpated in the scrotal sac. When one or both testes cannot be felt in the scrotum the baby should be examined again at 4–6 weeks of age, and again if necessary at three months. If descent has not taken place, referral to a consultant surgeon is made so that appropriate treatment can be instituted without delay. This usually involves an operation to replace the testes in the scrotal sac. Treatment of the undescended testes is important because:

1 It will increase the chances of satisfactory sperm production. The undescended testes will manufacture the male sex hormones and ensure normal sexual development, but the sperm-producing mechanism is impaired and, if the condition is bilateral, infertility results.
2 It results in a normal cosmetic appearance, preventing embarrassment particularly when school age is reached.
3 It reduces the risk of later malignant change to which the undescended testis is particularly liable.

Treatment should be carried out early, certainly before the age of five years, in order to achieve optimum results.

Circumcision Parents frequently seek advice about the need for circumcision. The foreskin is not fully retractable at birth in at least 90 % of boys but becomes so in the majority by four years of age. Circumcision is not indicated unless there is true phimosis or recurrent balanitis.

Skin

Naevi or birthmarks may be noted. The most common form is the red 'stork mark' which is found on the nape of the neck and the forehead, and disappears gradually. The capillary and cavernous naevi which arise from an abnormal collection of small blood vessels in the skin rarely need active treatment. The capillary naevi (strawberry birthmark) which appear shortly after birth grow very rapidly for about 12 months and then begin to regress spontaneously. The mother often needs continued reassurance that spontaneous resolution will indeed take place. Cavernous haemangioma (port wine stain), on the other hand, causes a permanent skin blemish which cannot yet be successfully treated in childhood, although developments in the laser techniques offer some hope for the future. Modern cosmetic aids may, in the meantime, help to conceal the disfigurement.

Nappy rash frequently occurs in normal babies and may be noted in routine examination, or more commonly it is a reason for consultation. Nappy rash may be caused by:

Ammoniacal dermatitis. The urea in the urine is broken down by contact with enzymes in the faeces to form ammonia, which irritates the napkin area of the skin. This is less likely to happen when the stools are acid, as in breast-fed babies. Advice is given regarding frequent nappy changing, washing of nappies in pure soap rather than detergents, with a final rinse of diluted vinegar, and protection of the skin by creams or silicone barrier preparations. Ammoniacal dermatitis can occur in babies whose general care is excellent, but a severe persistent form may be one sign of neglect.

Monilial infection. Thrush, more commonly associated with mouth infection, can also give rise to a nappy rash and should be considered particularly when a rash fails to respond to ordinary treatment. Swabs from the napkin area will show the presence of the *Candida* organisms. The treatment is the application of nystatin cream at each napkin change, and oral thrush should be dealt with at the same time by the use of nystatin oral suspension.

Seborrhoeic dermatitis. This shows a brownish-red scaly rash which appears not only in the napkin area but also in the skin in other areas of the body such as the scalp, behind the ears, the neck and axillae. A hydrocortisone cream, together with general measures as in ammoniacal dermatitis, is usually effective.

Eczema   This is an allergic condition although usually the precipitating cause is not known; it is less common in breast-fed babies. There is often a history of eczema, asthma or hay fever in other members of the family. Eczema often begins as a red patch on the face or in the creases of the limbs, but in severe cases can affect almost the whole body. It is extremely irritating and measures to prevent scratching, and possibly secondary infection, are important. Cortisone preparations applied locally are extremely valuable in keeping the condition under control.

The blood

Although haemoglobin estimation is not considered necessary as part of the routine physical examination of a child, the possibility of anaemia should be kept in mind when such symptoms as lethargy, poor appetite and disturbed sleep are mentioned by the parent. Pallor of the skin is an unreliable sign; inspection of the mucous membranes of the lower eyelid and of the lips is a better indication. Haemoglobin estimation confirms the diagnosis. Causes of anaemia include:

1   Iron deficiency, which is the commonest cause and is usually the result of a poor dietary intake.
2   Repeated infections or other chronic illnesses which can interfere with the absorption and utilisation of iron.

3   Genetic factors which, in some children of West Indian or African origin, give rise to sickle-cell anaemia (Chapter 8).
4   More rarely, lead poisoning and leukaemia.

Treatment of anaemia depends on its cause. Simple iron deficiency anaemia responds well to oral iron either in tablet or liquid form, and its recurrence is prevented by ensuring an adequate amount of iron-containing foods such as meat (particularly liver) and eggs.

Teeth

The times at which teeth erupt vary a great deal from child to child. On average, the first tooth (usually the lower central incisor) appears between the age of 6–10 months and the first dentition is complete by the age of three years. Occasionally a baby is born with one or more teeth and, at the other extreme, others do not have a tooth until after their first year. The majority of babies have very little trouble with teething, although in a few cases it may cause sore gums and some discomfort. Some parents tend to associate intercurrent illness such as bronchitis, diarrhoea and convulsions with teething, and so discount their risks. This is a dangerous practice and it should be explained to parents that delay in seeking advice for these conditions is unwise.

Past and future

The fact that the physical examination of every child at frequent intervals is no longer thought to be necessary is a reflection of the improvement in general health which has been achieved in the past hundred years. This contrasts with conditions at the beginning of the century when the incidence of chronic or recurrent illness, or established handicap, was such that repeated examination of all children was held in high priority. Increasingly successful techniques in the field of congenital heart surgery may call for earlier diagnosis than is possible from clinical examination, and screening by electrocardiographic examination at birth is a probability for the future. In other aspects of physical health, the main direction for the future seems to be in the field of prevention by the use of health education in enlarging parents' knowledge of their child's needs in specific aspects of general care and diet (including breast-feeding), in increasing their awareness of early warning signs of illness and the sources of help and advice available to them.

6

Surveillance of Health III

Development in the Early Years

The total development of a child at any age is the summation of changes taking place in several different fields:

1 Locomotion
2 Manipulation
3 Vision
4 Hearing
5 Speech
6 Social activity and behaviour

Surveillance follows progress in all of these aspects.

The central nervous system is the key system on which development primarily depends; it is the pathway through which stimuli from the environment are received, interpreted and translated into appropriate responses. Each child is an individual and develops at his own rate; quite striking variations may be found in the developmental achievements of different children of the same age, even amongst children of the same family. Surveillance of development is based on a knowledge of the range of ages within which it is normal for certain milestones (such as walking and talking) to be reached. Within this normal range, average ages of developmental achievement are useful guidelines but should not be applied as rigid criteria for the individual child. Developmental progress, if not average, may well be within the limits of the normal range. Parents frequently use average ages with which to compare the development of one child with another, and much needless worry can be avoided by helping them understand the concept of the range of normal.

Times of screening

Development implies change and surveillance involves a series of assessments at different times from birth onwards by which overall development relative to age can be checked. The neo-natal assessment includes an examination of the central nervous system, with particular regard to reflexes characteristic of the newborn, and forms a base-line for future reference. Following this, ages can be selected which take into account the average times at which important features of development can usefully be observed. Although ages are chosen when screening will be most profitable, an experienced doctor or health visitor is able to make a check of development in a child of any age who may be seen primarily for another purpose such as immunisation. Staff involved in developmental surveillance need a knowledge of normal child development and simple techniques by which progress can be measured, together with a realisation of the importance of assessing the child as a whole. Referral is made to a paediatrician or multidisciplinary team (Chapter 10) for more detailed assessment when development appears to be significantly delayed.

It is useful to consider the progression of events in each aspect of development, together with some reasons as to why delay might occur.

Locomotion

Each child passes through a succession of changes, starting with the development of head control, until he is finally able to walk unaided. These changes are noted by observing the child's posture and activities in different positions, and include for example:

Sitting for a short time without support	9 months
Pulling up to stand	9 months
Walking holding on to furniture	10–11 months
Crawling	10 months
Walking unaided	13 months

The development of walking is encouraged by giving the child opportunities to sit, stand and move about freely. Although the average age at which walking unaided begins is 13 months, some children will be able to do so as early as 8 months whilst others, quite normal in development, do not walk until two years of age. Delay in walking may be due to:

1 Muscles that are too rigid or too flabby—such as occurs in cerebral palsy (page 203) and spina bifida (page 201)
2 Lack of opportunity and practice
3 Mental retardation (page 202)
4 Familial tendency
5 Shuffling as an easy alternative method of getting about.

A child not walking by the age of two years is usually referred for specialist advice. Once independent walking has been achieved the child develops, over the next three or four years, the increasing ability to maintain balance and co-ordinate movements as seen for example in

Running	2 years
Climbing	2½–3 years
Jumping	3 years
Standing on one leg	3 years
Hopping	4 years
Skipping	5 years

Manipulation

A remarkable series of changes take place in the first year of life in the field of manipulation. The newborn baby cannot purposefully hold any object in his hand, but by the average age of 10 months he can co-ordinate fine movements and vision so as to pick up and hold, between the thumb and index finger, a small object like a pellet of paper placed on the table in front of him. This is an important developmental landmark. In the intervening months, purposeful grasping has gradually developed through the stages of:

Holding a rattle placed in the hand	4 months
Reaching out for, and grasping, a toy	6 months
Transferring a cube from hand to hand, using first the whole palm to grasp and hold	6 months
Refining movements to the pincer grasp	10 months

Speed and precision in manipulation follow in the next 3–4 years, so that the child becomes able to perform quite elaborate tasks which involve a complex series of co-ordinated movement of hands and fingers. Simple tests with play material show, for example, his ability to:

Build towers of cubes of increasing heights	from 18 months onwards
Thread beads on a shoelace	3 years
Hold a pencil in an adult way	3 years

Manipulative skills are encouraged by the provision of play material which does not necessarily have to include expensive or elaborate toys. A little ingenuity can convert many household articles into enjoyable and educational playthings.

Difficulties in the field of manipulation needing further investigation include abnormality of grasp and lack of co-ordination relative to age. They may arise because of:

1   Mental retardation (page 202)
2   Cerebral palsy (page 203)
3   Lack of opportunity and practice, particularly when provision of play material is inadequate

Vision

Screening tests indicate whether visual function is developing normally or whether there are any defects which need investigation. The type of test varies with the age of the child.

Early observation

The ability of the baby to fix his gaze on near objects develops during the first six weeks and the intent way in which the infant watches his mother's face is a valuable observation:

1 Tests using a ball dangling on a piece of string about 12 inches (30 cm) away from the baby's face demonstrate his increasing ability to follow a moving object in all directions by the age of six months.
2 The location of a small pellet of paper as used in testing manipulative skills gives an indication of near vision at 10 months.
3 The child will watch a small toy being pulled across the room 10 feet (3 metres) away from him at one year.

From this age, more refined testing can be done and each eye can be tested in turn:

4 From the age of two years the Stycar miniature toy test can be used; this involves the identification, at a distance of 10 feet, of small toys carefully selected for size and shape.
5 The Stycar test types can be used from 3 years onwards to test visual acuity through the recognition and matching of the shapes of selected letters of different sizes.
6 Near vision can be tested at 3 years by watching the child pick up one strand of 'hundreds and thousands' placed on the observer's palm.

In addition to screening for visual acuity, it is also essential to test children for squint.

Squint (strabismus)   At birth, both eyes move independently. In the first six months they gradually start functioning together so as to focus simultaneously on an object. If this does not occur, a squint is present which, if not corrected, may lead to impairment of vision in the squinting eye. Two simple tests are commonly used to detect a squint:

1 *The cover test.* The eyes fix on an object such as a pencil held (a) 1 foot (30 cm) and (b) 6 feet (180 cm) away from the face. During fixation one eye is covered with the hand or a light patch; any movement in the uncovered eye denotes a squint. When the covered eye is uncovered, note is taken of movement in that eye which indicates a latent squint.
2 *The reflected light test.*   A small light is held about 1 foot (30 cm) away from the child's face. Normally there is a symmetrical reflection of the light in the centre of both pupils. In a squinting eye, the symmetry is disturbed.

Screening for squint can be carried out by doctors or health visitors or, alternatively, by orthoptists who have a wide range of equipment at their disposal.

Treatment. Any child over the age of six months with a suspected or overt squint should be referred to a consultant ophthalmology unit as treatment at an early stage enables satisfactory vision to be established in the squinting eye. The exact type of treatment varies with the individual child and may include:

1 The wearing of glasses
2 Occlusion of the non-squinting eye
3 Orthoptic exercises

In a small proportion of cases, squint may be a sign of an underlying serious condition and prompt referral enables an early diagnosis to be made.

Visual handicap

Common forms of visual defects such as squint, and short- and long-sightedness are correctable by appropriate treatment or prescription of glasses. A few children have severe visual handicap resulting from, for example, inherited conditions such as retinoblastoma or from rubella infection during pregnancy, and need special help from an early age. The parents, too, need support and practical advice to enable them to accept their child's disability and help him to become independent. Many education departments employ support teachers who visit the home and help in parent counselling, discussing ways in which other aspects of development can be encouraged, and advising on educational provisions. The Royal National Institute for the Blind (RNIB) provides home visitors to assist parents in any difficulties they may be experiencing.

Tests of vision

1 Screening tests from 6 weeks onwards
2 Specific tests for squint

Hearing

Early ascertainment that hearing is normal is an important aspect of developmental screening. Early diagnosis of deafness:

1 Enables training for speech to be given by home teachers and speech therapists during the important early years of learning. Parents are

helped to understand ways in which the child's general development can be encouraged and the importance of vision in the understanding of things normally associated with sound, particularly in watching facial movements and expressions during speech. Some children may benefit from wearing a hearing aid from an early age; models are becoming more effective and easier for the very young child to accept.

2   Enables formal education to be planned. Some deaf children will be helped in speech and general development by attendance at a nursery class.

3   Alerts one to the possibility of other defects being present.

Hearing tests

It is recognised that simple tests of hearing are most easily performed between the ages of six to nine months, by which time the baby is developing the ability to localise sounds. Testing can be done in the home or wherever quiet surroundings are possible. The tests involve observation of the child's response to a variety of sounds including the human voice, a spoon moved gently round the inside of a cup, and high- and low-pitched rattles. The sounds are made to each side of the child, about 18 inches (45 cm) away and at ear level, making sure that the tester is out of sight. A baby of six to nine months with normal hearing will turn his head promptly towards the origin of the sound. The few who fail to respond in a second screening are referred for more specialised examination at an audiology clinic. Every effort is made to ensure that all children are tested, particularly those at increased risk, for example where there is a family incidence, a history of maternal rubella during pregnancy, prematurity, jaundice, or ear infection.

An examination of hearing for speech is recommended for all children between the ages of $2\frac{1}{2}$–3 years. The screening tests at this age are based on the identification of selected toys (Stycar Toys Test) or objects in a picture named by the examiner.

As well as specific screening tests, other observations, particularly on the part of the mother, may lead to a suspicion that hearing is not normal:

1   A baby under three months of age who does not respond to a sudden loud noise by blinking or 'startle' movements.

2   A baby of seven months not responding to his name.

3   Little progress in early speech development (6–12 months) or a later marked delay or deficiency in speech.

4   An older child may express his frustration in not being able to communicate satisfactorily in behaviour disturbances such as temper tantrums, withdrawal, or head banging.

```
        Ascertainment of hearing
   1  Screening tests at 6–9 months
   2  Further tests at 2½–3 years
   3  Clinical observation
```

Speech and language

A baby is born with the ability to make sounds (vocalisation). From four months, vowels and consonants join to form syllables which, from the age of seven months, are repeated constantly (babbling). The baby goes on to imitate sounds which he hears around him, in words spoken frequently and repetitively. It is very important for a mother to talk to her baby from the beginning; he may not understand what she says in actual words, but sounds, intonations and rhythms all stimulate the development of speech. Understanding of the meaning of words is achieved by the mother constantly linking the sight or sound of an object with its name. Many children at the age of a year are able to say two or three words with meaning. Words are put together to form simple phrases from eighteen months, and sentences from the average age of two years. During this period, many sounds are produced resembling speech but which are quite unintelligible (jargon). In the course of the next few years, a child's vocabulary increases rapidly from around fifty words at two years to over two thousand at five years. During this time he constantly questions and develops the ability to express actions, concepts of self and others and abstract ideas in speech.

```
                    Development of speech
   1  Babbling                            7–8   months
   2  First word with meaning            12–14 months
   3  Sequences of two-three words       18–24 months
   4  Normal speech                       3–3½ years
```

Children vary a great deal in the rate at which speech develops, some speaking fluently by eighteen months or even earlier, others remaining relatively silent until the age of four. Concern is felt when a child of 18 months is not saying one or two words.

The use of speech in language and the development of understanding are as important to assess as the ability to say words. A child should respond to his name by the age of twelve months and understand simple requests by eighteen months. During the third and following years, assessment is made of the ability to name and identify familiar objects, put labels to actions and describe pictures. Spontaneous speech is noted, and inability to use phrases of 2–3 words in a child of three is an indication for further investigation. When speech is delayed referral is made to a paediatrician who may then involve a speech therapist. The following more common causes may be considered:

1 *Deafness.* A child who is deaf cannot imitate sounds which he does not hear. Effective screening procedures should detect deafness at an early age, but any child with significant speech delay should be re-tested.
2 *Mental retardation.* Delay in speech is frequently marked. The delay is not only in the saying of words, but in comprehension of their meaning, and the use of speech in language (page 202).
3 *Lack of stimulation.* Emotionally deprived children and those who do not hear a great deal of speech may show delay.
4 *Family history.* Other members of the family may have shown similar delay.
5 *Autism.* Delay or regression in speech may be a sign of autism.

Disturbances of Speech

Some children, whilst not essentially showing true delay in developing speech, show some difficulty in achieving fluency.

Indistinct speech (Dyslalia) All children pass through a phase when their speech is indistinct, but in some this persists and the child may be faced with difficulty and embarrassment on school entry. The hearing should be tested and speech therapy is indicated.

Stammer Repetition of a syllable or a whole word frequently occurs as a normal phase of speech development but in some children this is prolonged and parents become worried about its persistence. Much can be done by reassuring the parents, encouraging them to adopt simple ways of helping such as not drawing attention to the hesitancy, speaking clearly themselves, suggesting the child's participation in reading stories, and by resolving any anxiety or stress. Speech therapy is advised when, in spite of simple measures, the stammer persists.

Social activity and behaviour

Social development progresses as a result of a wide range of changes through which the child learns to live contentedly with himself as an individual within society. In order to do this, he must acquire increasing degrees of independence and confidence in himself, and come to recognise the rights of other people.

Independence and social skills

Throughout infancy, childhood and adolescence, skills are acquired which transform the helpless baby into an independent adult. In the early years, the child learns to use his powers of mobility, manipulation, vision and hearing to perform activities of daily living. He learns to:

feed himself with a spoon	13 months
drink from a cup without much spilling	15 months
put on shoes and socks and simple dressing	2 years
manage buttons	3–4 years
tie shoelaces	5 years
washes hands and face	5 years

The ability to achieve tasks, however small, gives the child increasing confidence in himself and encourages self-reliance.

Relationships

It is in the field of relationships that social activities and behaviour become so closely interlinked. Initially, the young baby's world consists almost entirely of his mother. He is completely dependent on her for the essentials of existence and has to learn how best to make his needs known and understood. He learns how to communicate long before actual speech develops, by a variety of sounds, expressions and gestures, and is helped by his mother's reciprocal communication in expression, words, contact and action. His first social smile appears at about five to six weeks. He begins to recognise other people within the family circle and demonstrates affection, but from 7 to 18 months or so shows a wariness with strangers and the emotional need of a familiar person nearby.

Gradually, the acceptable norms of behaviour are learned through recognition of signs of approval and disapproval on the part of others, particularly parents. The young child becomes increasingly aware of himself as a person in relation to a widening circle of people around him and experiences the conflict that can arise in attempting to find the balance between immediate gratification of his own wishes and the need to win the approval of others. He learns how to control his aggression and self-assertion and responds to encouragement and praise. It is in these aspects of development that the relationship between parents and child is so important and, as in other fields, parents need to be aware of how they can help. From the earliest days, the provision of a loving environment and a framework of consistency give the child the sense of a warm secure world whose limits he knows, within which he may experiment and test and from which he may gradually expand his horizons. Special difficulty is often found in the establishment of good social relationships where there are adverse circumstances such as broken homes, marital discord, maternal depression or unwanted pregnancies.

Screening of social development

Some aspects of social development are not capable of being screened in the precise way possible in other fields, but assessment can be made during routine surveillance examinations, observation of play and discussion with parents.

Surveillance examinations The routine surveillance of other fields of development often gives information about social development, for example, manipulative skills in tasks of daily living, the use of speech for communication and the understanding of simple requests. Observation of the mother-child interaction will illustrate the social responses of smiling, showing affection, attitudes to strangers and the ability to tolerate varying periods of separation. The parents' own comments on their child's progress give important information on aspects which cannot always be quickly and simply observed in a test situation, such as dressing himself, and bowel and bladder control. Their observations may also give some indications of their expectations of the child in relation to his age.

Observations of play This is very rewarding where social developments are concerned. Play is necessary from the beginning of life (Fig. 6.1).

1   A child learns through play in all its forms, whether it be with toys, imitative play in household activities, or in the company of other children. Through play, a child learns about size, shape, weight, texture, colour, position and movement. He discovers ways in which he can use his body to move, think and fashion with increasing co-ordination and control. Difficulties in locomotion, manipulation, hearing, vision or unusually obsessive play with one toy may become apparent in observation of play.

2   Sociability is encouraged through play with other children from the age of 2–3 years. Observations of a child in a group of others of the same age will give indications of his ability to mix, share and work out arguments and disagreements.

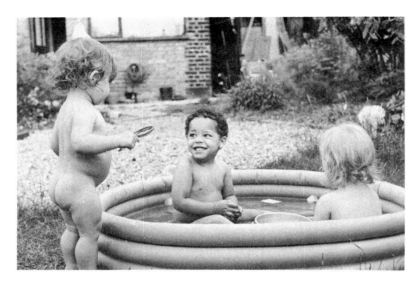

Fig. 6.1 Play helps development (Photograph courtesy of Vanessa Mitchell)

3 Children also use play as a safety-valve for stress. Feelings which they cannot or dare not express openly, such as aggression or jealousy, may be channelled acceptably through play, and a trained observer can appreciate the significance of different play situations.

4 Play allows children to give their imagination full rein, and acts as an early preparation for real-life situations.

Discussion of parental concern Parents frequently express doubt or concern about some aspect of their child's social development and behaviour. Their observations help in the assessment of the child's development, and they in their turn find it valuable to discuss matters with a doctor or health visitor. Some of the more common situations involve such everyday activities as feeding, sleeping or toileting. The majority of children at some time or another have phases of 'awkwardness' which in most instances are temporary and, if handled in the right way, resolve happily. Discussion, explanation and reassurance help parents to avoid a perpetuation of the situation and lessen the risk of tension between themselves and their child.

Feeding difficulties. These arise particularly with the toddler and, all too often, concern on the part of the mother and assertion of self by the child can result in a battle of wills. Explanation of the situation, reassurance of fears of under-eating and advice on management can resolve difficulties at an early stage and prevent a more intractable situation developing.

Sleeping problems. The sleep needs of individual children vary a great deal. Concern may be expressed about the child who sleeps very little or whose sleep (and that of the family) is broken. Discussion with the doctor or health visitors could suggest ways in which the period of potential strain could be relieved.

Temper tantrums. These are a natural occurrence in the child of two or three years who finds his intentions thwarted and is unable at his stage of development to control his feelings in a mature way. Parents can be helped to understand this and advised not only on how to deal with the actual outburst, but also in ways of forestalling the issue.

Jealousy. This often occurs when a new baby arrives in the household and can show itself in different ways, ranging from aggressive behaviour to regression into more infantile habits of feeding or loss of bladder control. Awareness of the possibility helps parents to appreciate the need for the older child to have periods of individual attention and to understand the significance of any behaviour disturbance.

Toilet training. Simple discussion of the ways in which bladder control is achieved is helpful, particularly in encouraging the mother to respond appropriately to signals from the child rather than adopting a rigid training programme. The majority of children are dry during the day by the end of the third year, having passed through the sequence of telling the mother (1) when their pants are wet, (2) just before urine is passed, but too late, and (3) in time. The age of dryness at night is more variable—75 % will achieve this by three years of age, 90 % by five years. For some parents, the fact that the child of three is still wetting the bed becomes a matter of anxiety which may hinder, rather than help, the situation. Reassurance can be given that in some children, control is not achieved for another year or two and the great majority become dry spontaneously.

Established behaviour disturbance Serious disturbances such as severe aggression, withdrawal, prolonged head-banging and rocking may be the result of a difficult parent-child relationship and indicate the need for special help from a child psychologist or psychiatrist.

Multiple developmental delay In some children, screening will detect a specific delay in a single aspect of development such as hearing. In others, delay or abnormal patterns of development become apparent in more than one field. The combined effect of several defects can lead to many problems throughout the child's life. Early detection, whilst not always leading to a cure in the accepted sense of the term, enables therapy and management to be introduced so as to allow the child's potential to develop as far as it can.

> ### *Screening for social development*
>
> 1 Surveillance in other fields of development such as manipulation and speech
> 2 Observation of play
> 3 Discussions with parents

Achievements and the future

Improvements in ante-natal and peri-natal care have helped to ensure a potential for normal development in the majority of children. In the last 20 years, programmes of surveillance have changed from those directed mainly towards children whose history appeared to place them at increased risk of developmental delay, to those attempting to screen the total child population; the effectiveness of the latter is now in the process of evaluation. One problem which has still to be satisfactorily resolved is that of reaching all children, particularly those whose social circumstances place them in most need of surveillance. These are the children where developmental delay is often due to lack of stimulus and opportunity rather than to pathological conditions, and where parent education and direction towards playgroups, nursery classes and toy libraries could greatly change the picture. Further improvements in developmental surveillance could result from more effective means of screening. This is particularly the case in the detection of deafness where methods of identification soon after birth are available but not yet in such a form that would seem to make their general application economically practicable.

7

Surveillance of Health IV

School Children

Good health in its broadest sense is needed to enable children to accept and respond fully to the opportunities and challenges of school life. Ill-health, handicap, and social and emotional difficulties may result in frequent absences from school, lack of concentration, or an inability to absorb, understand and utilise all the new and varied concepts with which the child is presented. The programme of surveillance has special importance in relation to the child's capacity to benefit from education; it also makes its own educational contribution in encouraging the child to understand his body and to accept increasing responsibility for his own future health (Fig. 7.1).

Programmes of surveillance are usually carried out by the school doctor and school nurse, who should be familiar with the principles of educational health. Discussions with parent and teacher regarding health and educational progress, and a knowledge of the child's home background are essential in building up a complete picture. Other professionals such as the general practitioner, the psychologist and speech therapist may have important contributions to make and, at times, referral for consultant paediatric advice is indicated.

The start of school health surveillance is a comprehensive examination at or around the time of primary school entry. This includes:

1 A review of past health and development, including discussion with parent and teacher.
2 Measurement of height and weight.
3 A physical examination.
4 Simple screening of neurological development to detect any abnormal functioning of the central nervous system whcih may foreshadow or account for difficulties in learning.
5 Screening of vision and hearing.

Following the initial examination, which forms a baseline for future reference, it is not now considered necessary to examine every child again during school life, but rather to select those children where further examination is indicated. This procedure would include those children for whom:

1 The first examination has shown a need for follow-up.
2 There is concern on the part of parent or teacher about the child's health.

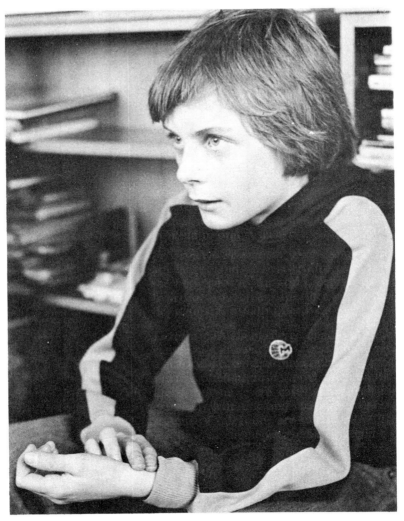

Fig. 7.1 Surveillance of health! *Colin New*

3 Answers to a health questionnaire completed by parents suggest a health problem.
4 Scrutiny of attendance records shows repeated absences from school.

In addition, regular measurements of growth and tests of vision and hearing should be carried out on every child. The school nurse holds sessions for personal hygiene inspection and may take the opportunity to watch children during physical education classes, so as to observe general activity, motor skills and co-ordination. It is recommended that every child between the ages of 13–14 years should have an interview with the school doctor to give the opportunity for discussion on health or related matters.

Surveillance of school children

1 Initial school entry examination
2 Subsequent selective examination
3 Interview with 13–14 year old children
4 Regular check of growth, vision and hearing
5 Observations by parent, teacher, school nurse or other professional workers

---

Surveillance is considered in detail under four headings:

1 Observation of growth
2 Physical examination and screening procedures
3 Developmental progress: learning, behavioural and social aspects
4 Scrutiny of attendance records

Observation of growth

Between the ages of 5–9 years, growth usually progresses steadily, but regular checks are recommended for every child during the primary school period to detect variations considered to be outside the range of normal. In older age groups measurements of height and weight can be reviewed for selected children. Growth is recorded on percentile charts.

1 The detection of short stature remains important, particularly when it is thought to be psycho-social in origin or due to primary growth hormone deficiency.

2 Normal variations in growth at the time of puberty may give rise to anxiety in some children. The spurt of growth and appearance of secondary sex characteristics occur within a wide range of years (9–14) and this may need explanation to the child. In a small proportion of boys, puberty is delayed and its accompanying growth changes, particularly in height, are late in appearing. This can be a source of worry to the boy and his parents; explanation and discussion will help to reassure them.

3 It is increasingly important to detect those children whose growth is adversely affected by an insufficient or poorly balanced diet resulting from financial difficulties in the family, so that help can be offered in the form of free milk and free school meals. The problems of weight loss due to anorexia nervosa is discussed later in the chapter.

4 Obesity remain a common problem. Detection in the early stages enables patterns of diet to be recommended which are more easily accepted because they do not need to be extreme. Health education for parents and children can help them to understand some of the factors leading to obesity, and the positive contribution to health which a balanced diet makes. Successful treatment of established obesity calls for great motivation and discipline on the part of parents and child in order to maintain, perhaps indefinitely, some modification of dietary habits. Sometimes an emotional difficulty underlies obesity, particularly during adolescence, and calls for counselling and therapy. Prescription of a suitable diet is reinforced by:
(a) Explanation and discussion with parent and child
(b) Regular weight checks
(c) Sympathetic listening to problems
(d) Encouragement of effort
(e) Praise for achievement of weight loss, however small
(f) Regular exercise.
Mutual support groups for older children on the lines of the adult 'Weight-Watchers' may be very valuable in helping to turn the problem into a shared one, rather than one which isolates them from their peers.

Surveillance of growth

1 Measurement of height to detect abnormally short stature
2 Measurement of weight to detect abnormally small weight gain and obesity

---

Physical examination and screening procedures

By the time a child reaches school-age, any physical problems arising from congenital abnormality should already have been detected. The physical examination on school entry is largely one of a confirmatory nature, but also includes simple tests of neurological development. Subsequent selective examinations will deal with any health problems brought forward by parent, teacher or child, either directly or by the health questionnaire. Many children with handicap or chronic illness such as asthma, diabetes or epilepsy, are educated in ordinary schools but their health and progress need regular monitoring. Their total surveillance will require the co-ordination of the findings and opinions of other professionals involved in their care (Chapters 9 and 10).

Screening procedures

Vision   On school entry it is important, particularly from the educational aspect, to screen the vision of every child to establish the adequacy of distant and near vision. Testing should be repeated at two-yearly intervals throughout school life to detect any difficulty in seeing, with referral for correction with glasses. Stycar test types, Keystone machine and Snellen test cards are used according to age.

Colour vision   The ability to distinguish and name colours should be established by the age of five. Some children have colour blindness and are unable to distinguish different colours, most commonly red from green. This can lead to difficulties at school when educational teaching methods involve the extensive use of colour apparatus, and can also influence the eventual choice of a career. Colour blindness is an inherited condition, more common in boys than girls, but all children should be screened using special Ishihara test cards at some time during their early primary school life.

Hearing   With efficient early screening tests for deafness, it is assumed that children with congenital deafness will have been identified long before they enter primary school. Screening of hearing is needed during school life to detect those children with a hearing loss due to other factors. Picture vocabulary or word tests are used on school entry, and screening by audiometry is carried out during the first or second years of school life. In addition, a teacher may refer a child for a hearing test at any time if deafness is suspected as a cause of educational difficulty. The most common test is called the 'sweep test' and is usually carried out by a school nurse with special training or an audiometrician. Children with an unsatisfactory test result are referred to an audiology clinic for further investigations.

A common cause of deafness in school children is the impairment of middle ear function due to an accumulation of a serous effusion ('glue-ear'). This produces a variable degree of deafness, usually less profound than that of congenital origin, but sufficient to produce educational and emotional problems if remaining untreated. 'Glue-ear' may respond to medical treatment designed to liquefy the secretion or may require surgery involving the incision of the ear drum in order to withdraw the accumulated serous fluid in the middle ear and the insertion of a fine plastic tube called a grommet which allows ventilation of the middle ear cavity. 'Glue-ear' may follow previous chronic otitis media.

Scoliosis A simple screening test at yearly intervals to detect adolescent scoliosis (lateral curvature of the spine) is recommended between the ages of 10–14 years, a time of rapid growth. If undetected, it may result in a permanent and unsightly spinal deformity which, in extreme cases, leads to distortion of the thoracic cage with subsequent respiratory distress. The test can be carried out by the school nurse. The child is asked to bend forward with the arms down and the palms together. Any asymmetry of the thoracic cage can be seen and referral made to an orthopaedic consultant. The treatment depends on the degree of scoliosis. Minor curvature may need nothing more than careful observation. More marked degrees are treated by some form of corset and brace which is worn consistently until sexual maturity. Severe curvature may need surgical correction. Other methods of treatment are being reviewed, particularly that of stimulating the muscles on the convex side of the curvature by electrodes implanted on or just under the skin. Adolescent scoliosis is much more common in girls and, when staff resources are limtied, they may be allotted screening priority.

Surveillance of physical health

1 Physical examination
2 Screening tests of: vision
                        hearing
                        scoliosis

Developmental progress: learning, behavioural, and social aspects

Statutory schooling covers a wide age-span, and children in different age groups show very different characteristics. Two major groups will be considered—5–9 years and 10 years onwards.

Children aged 5–9 years

During this period there are no major landmarks in development such as those which characterise the very early years of life. This is, rather, a period of steady progress when the developmental skills already achieved are refined and made more precise. The young child entering primary school spends a considerable period of the day away from home, so social and emotional adjustments are necessary. New relationships are made with adults; the child gains a widening circle of friends and needs to feel accepted as one of the group. During these years, parents or teachers may bring forward various aspects of a child's developmental progress for discussion with the school doctor.

Enuresis   This is the term used to describe lack of bladder control after the age of five; it most commonly occurs during sleep. Enuresis can present a distressing problem for parent and child alike. It can lead to anxiety on the part of the child, teasing from siblings, difficulties with holidays and additional work for the mother. It is probable that more than one factor may contribute to delayed bladder control:

1   There is sometimes a family history which indicates a genetically-determined lateness in maturation of bladder function.
2   Some children have an unusually small bladder and strong muscular contractions which together cause urgent emptying.
3   In other children, stress appears to be a factor particularly when control has previous been established and has later broken down.
4   Difficult environmental circumstances such as family discord or a broken home, especially if accompanied by lack of training at the appropriate age, may be the underlying cause.
5   In a very small number of children, organic causes are present, such as persistent urinary infection, undetected diabetes, spina bifida occulta, and ectopic opening of the urethra.

The successful management of enuresis is based on a sympathetic appreciation of the difficulties of parent and child, together with reassurance as to the eventual positive outcome and practical suggestions to relieve the immediate situation. A physical examination, including urine analysis, will exclude specific lesions. Advice includes:

1   Helping the parents adopt an attitude which is encouraging, non-punitive and matter-of-fact. At no time should they make the child feel he is not loved or cannot be helped.
2   Discussion of any episode of stress and ways of relief.
3   Practical suggestions regarding warmth at night, mattress protection and night-lights. Fluids should be taken freely during the day and the child encouraged to hold urine for as long as possible.
4   Adopting a system of marking dry nights with a star on a calander. Some children respond well to this, as it helps to build up their confidence and gives them a sense of achievement.
5   Using an electric alarm, which often works very well with children over the age of seven. The alarm is triggered off by a very small amount of urine wetting a pad placed under the sheet. The noise wakes the child, he gets up to turn off the alarm and goes to pass urine. After some time, the child will wake up before the bell rings or

may sleep through the night without passing urine. This method
involves understanding and co-operation from the child and parent.
6 The use of drugs to control enuresis, particularly imipramine, (more
commonly used as an anti-depressant). There is a tendency to relapse
once the drug is discontinued and, in some children, unpleasant side-
effects have been noticed.

Treatment of enuresis

1 Support and advice for parent and child
2 Some children respond to a 'star calender'
3 Children over seven often respond well to the electric
   buzzer
4 Drugs are not usually indicated

The 'clumsy child'   Children differ widely in their motor skills, but a
small group show a lack of muscle co-ordination which is outside the
normal range for their age. Their movements are clumsy, particularly
where speed, accuracy and precision are needed. They find difficulty in
running, hopping, catching a ball, writing and tying shoelaces, and may
be labelled as 'naughty' or 'not trying'. Some clumsy children are simply
late in maturing but in others a mild brain dysfunction or other
pathological condition underlies their difficulties. The school doctor
may refer for further neurological assessment and therapy, and will help
parents and teachers to appreciate the child's difficulties so that they can
encourage him to perform well within the limits of his ability.

The hyperactive child   Parents and teachers may complain that a child is
abnormally active in the sense that he is never still but his activity seems
without purpose, he has little concentration and is unresponsive to
discipline. Hyperactivity may be due to a variety of causes; some
children have underlying neurological disorders, some are mentally
retarded and in others the condition arises from emotional disturbances
associated with difficult home circumstances. Parents and teachers need
advice and support in the management of a hyperactive child, and in the
provision of an environment which gives sufficient interest and stimulation. Psychiatric help may be indicated and some children respond to
specific drug therapy to enable them to become more responsive to
teaching.

The child with learning difficulties   A small proportion of children
encounter difficulties in learning—a term which covers a wide range of
problems with an equally wide range of underlying factors. Previous
examinations may have identified a mentally retarded child or one

deprived of stimulation; these are children whose general level of performance is expectedly below average. Other children with average intelligence may fail to reach the expected standard of achievement because of a difficult home background or emotional stress. The neurological tests of the school entry examination may suggest that difficulties in learning in specific subjects, particularly reading (dyslexia), may be encountered. In other instances, parents or teachers are worried that a child is not progressing as well as they think he should. In any case of learning difficulty it is important, from the medical aspect, that vision and hearing are checked and that contributory conditions are identified. Educational psychologists and remedial teachers have special knowledge about ways in which the individual child may be helped.

The child with behaviour difficulties Behaviour difficulties may be brought to the school doctor's notice by parent, teacher or school nurse. Children's early behaviour is learned largely at home from the pattern which parents set for them. The majority of parents are able to give their child security based on love, affection, and a clear consistent framework of behaviour patterns and discipline which enables the child to adjust happily to school life. However, the personality of a child may be such that for a time, at least, school presents changes which give rise to continued stress. A reversion to bedwetting may occur in a child who had previously been dry. Sometimes, hidden anxiety is expressed in physical terms such as sleeping problems, lack of appetite, nausea, abdominal pain and headache. Sympathetic discussion with the parents can enable them to understand the difficulty, suggest ways of dealing with it and reassure them as to the eventual resolution.

The child with educational under-achievement due to learning difficulties, the bored gifted child, or the child who feels he is failing to live up to high parental expectations may express his distress in terms of unacceptable behaviour. In some families no consistently clear model for behaviour has been presented to the child—he may have lived, or still be living, in an atmosphere of domestic strife, marital discord, broken home, psychiatric illness in a parent, or have experienced rejection or frequent periods of separation from his mother or father. Consequently, behaviour difficulties arise such as aggression, disobedience, disruption of the class, persistent lying and stealing; other children become withdrawn and tend to be overlooked because they cause no trouble.

An appreciation of the roots of the problem is essential if adequate help is to be given. Management involves a recognition and improvement, as far as possible, of the whole family situation rather than attempting to deal with the child in isolation. It may require the resources not only of the school health service, but the general practitioner, social worker, educational welfare officer, the school psychological service and the child psychiatrist.

Situations likely to cause behaviour difficulties

1 Stress
2 Undetected or unresolved learning difficulties
3 Boredom
4 Unrealistic parental expectations
5 Disturbed family environment

Surveillance of development in children 5–9 years may reveal:

1 The child with enuresis
2 The 'clumsy child'
3 The hyperactive child
4 The child with learning difficulties
5 The child with behaviour difficulties

Children from 10 years upwards

From the age of 10 years (or in some children a little earlier) a new phase of development emerges with the rapidly occurring changes associated with adolescence. This is a period of transition from childhood to adulthood characterised by physical changes, the maturation of the sexual organs, the emergence of sexual feelings, and the desire for independence which often conflicts with the reality of dependence on parents and the retention of the security of home. Most adolescents gradually adjust to this period of rapid change. In a few, social and emotional problems become evident, some arising for the first time during the period of adolescence, others as a continuation or recurrence of earlier behaviour difficulties.

It is not always easy for the adolescent to express his feelings or to find the right person in whom to confide. Within his school environment, a school counsellor or one of the health service staff may be the appropriate person. The doctor and school nurse should be regarded as part of the school counselling service, and self-referral to them should be accepted as a desirable practice. It is recommended that all children between the ages of 13–14 should have an opportunity for private discussion with the school doctor when matters relating to health, general development and relationships could be raised. Such an interview would enable reassurance to be given and responsibility for future health discussed; problems needing resolution might be revealed. Medical examination may be indicated in a proportion of children or referral to agencies equipped to give appropriate help can be made. Early identification of potential problems and of contributory factors in home or school life may prevent serious trouble arising.

Surveillance of social and emotional health in adolescence

Problems may be recognised from:

1 Interviews with 13–14 year old children
2 Self-referral to doctor or nurse
3 Counselling within the school
4 Concern by parents or teacher

Problems associated with adolescence include:

1 Anti-social behaviour Many adolescents have periods of disobedience, flaunting of authority, unruly or aggressive behaviour which form part of their struggle to achieve independence and identity as an individual. It is often difficult to define what is essentially a transient phase of adolescence and what constitutes abnormal behaviour. Adolescents showing persistent lying, stealing, violence and other forms of behaviour which go beyond the limits of acceptability, will need help from a pool of people including the school health service, family doctor, school psychological service, child psychiatrist and social worker. At all times the home background and the problems and needs of the family as a whole are taken into consideration.

2 Social problems During adolescence, problems may arise in connection with the use of alcohol and drugs. These will be discussed (along with smoking) in Chapter 8.

3 Sexual problems Earlier maturation means many children are sexually developed at an age when their capacity to appreciate and cope with the emotional aspects of relationship has not yet reached a corresponding degree of maturity. This, together with the more permissive attitude of society today, has resulted in many adolescents experimenting with sex. This may result in pregnancy and, where promiscuity is a feature, to the risk of contracting a sexually-transmitted disease. The health education aspect of sexual problems is discussed in Chapter 8.

School girl pregnancy. About 5000 girls under the age of 16 become pregnant each year, and approximately two-thirds of the pregnancies are terminated. The pregnant school girl needs the professional skills of medical, nursing and social work staff. Early attendance for ante-natal care enables considered decisions to be made about continuation or termination of pregnancy, and ensures adequate supervision should it continue. Social workers help the girl and her parents to work through the difficult decision regarding the future of the baby and any deeper emotional problems which might underlie the situation. They also give practical advice regarding finance and accommodation. During pregnancy the girl may be able to continue at school for some time, or may receive home tuition or education in a special centre. It is important that she should have opportunities to discuss her future educational life in the light of the range of possibilities open to her. Should the decision be to keep the baby, the health visitor has a special task in helping the girl develop her capacity for mothering and accept her role in a realistic manner. Facilities for contraceptive advice should be made known and, where possible, referral made to centres specially equipped to deal with adolescents.

4   Psychiatric problems   Other disorders in adolescents include:

Anorexia nervosa. An increasingly common disturbance in adolescent girls, particularly those of higher intelligence and upper social class, is a refusal to eat sufficient food to maintain body weight. This is often accompanied by amenorrhea (absence of normal menstrual function). Anorexia nervosa is a complex disorder and, although appearing superficially to stem from an obsessive desire to be slim, may basically be associated with a deep-seated fear of growing into a mature woman. The treatment includes psychiatric help in the form of individual and family therapy, together with measures to restore physical health.

Suicide attempts. The increase in attempted suicide is also causing concern. Suicide attempts are more common in girls, and by far the most common form is taking an overdose of drugs such as aspirin. 'Attempt' does not mean a 'failed' suicide, but is rather a feature indicating feelings and difficulties which are unable to be expressed directly. Referral for appropriate psychotherapeutic help is indicated, which again will include not only treatment of the girl, but also family therapy.

Surveillance of adolescents may reveal:

1   Anti-social behaviour
2   Social problems e.g. alcohol and drugs
3   Sexual problems; school girl pregnancy
4   Anorexia nervosa
5   History of attempted suicide

Scrutiny of attendance records

Part of the surveillance programme of school children is that of scrutinising the attendance records to detect children who have frequent or prolonged absences from school. The most frequent cause is illness, particularly chronic illness. A small proportion of absences signify the classical truants—children who voluntarily absent themselves from school without the knowledge or permission of parents or teacher, finding (for them) more attractive alternatives to spending the day in the classroom. Another cause is school refusal.

School refusal This differs from truancy in that it is not a voluntarily chosen absence but an inability beyond the control of the child to attend school. Some children show increasing reluctance or absolutely refuse to set out for school; psychosomatic symptoms occur in others, such as vomiting, headache, abdominal pain and diarrhoea, severe enough to keep the child at home on school-days, but not occurring at the weekend. In yet others, a panic-stricken child may return home as soon as, or before, school is reached. School refusal can occur in all ages of children and is more common in children of average or above average intelligence, with no apparent educational difficulties.

Treatment for school refusal involves:

1 Recognition of the true nature of the condition.
2 Examination to exclude physical disease and to reassure parent and child.
3 Investigation into any fears of school the child may have, with appropriate adjustment where possible.
4 Investigation of any aspect of home life which is giving rise to acute anxiety in the child.
5 Referral to the child psychiatrist if modification of contributory factors at home or school does not improve the situation.

> *Scrutiny of school attendance*
>
> Absence may be due to:
>
> 1 Illness
> 2 Truancy
> 3 School refusal

Gifted children

Much attention is focussed on children showing developmental delay, but at the other end of the scale are those children whose progress and achievement in many fields is superior to those of the average child. Recognition of a truly gifted child is just as important as the identification of a child delayed in development, as he too has special needs to be met if his potential is to be achieved and the problems arising from isolation, boredom and frustration avoided.

Different education authorities adopt different measures to help their gifted children, varying from separate schools, ability-grouped classes, flexibility in age of admission and transfer from school to school.

The National Association for Gifted Children offers advice to parents and helps to promote special activity ventures on a day or residential basis which offer opportunities to extend and stimulate interests.

Present and future

Better standards of living, improved diet, and advances in medical diagnosis and treatment have all contributed greatly to the improved growth and health of school children since the beginning of the century. Screening of the total school population for selected conditions identifies those children with problems likely to interfere with their education or to affect adversely their future health. It is possible that in future other screening tests will be included; the value of measurement of blood pressure is currently being evaluated. Where development is concerned, the recognition of children with specific learning difficulties has led to appropriate help being made available, but more needs to be done to help the gifted child.

The majority of children pass through childhood and adolescence into adulthood without serious difficulty, but a proportion show social and behavioural problems which are causing concern both for the present and the future. Many of thier difficulties are related to circumstances in family life which, in turn, is influenced by the attitudes of present day society about marriage, divorce, sexual promiscuity and social practices; unemployment adds to the scene. Health, education and social services are acknowledging the value of a flexible but co-ordinated approach to these complex problems, the resolution of which involves tackling many different aspects of life today.

8
Health Education

The aim of health education is to teach people how to value health, explain ways in which good health can be promoted, and help in the understanding of the purpose and wise use of services. There are two main components in health education:

1 The promotion of factual, accurate and up-to-date information on health matters, presented in terms which are easily understood and acceptable.
2 The influencing of attitudes towards health and helping people make wise decisions based on the information which has been presented to them.

Health education
1 Gives factual, accurate and up-to-date information on health matters
2 Influences attitudes to health and helps people make wise decisions

---

The health educators

Responsibility for the promotion of health is shared by everybody, although certain people and groups have specific contributions to make:

1 The Health Education Council is responsible at national level for the promotion and development of health education.

2 A health education department staffed by health education officers and technical staff may serve one or more health districts. The health education officer is responsible for:

(a) Assisting the District Medical Officer to assess the health education needs of the district community.
(b) Developing appropriate health education programmes.
(c) Providing resource material—leaflets, posters, tapes, slides, films and exhibitions for professional and public use.
(d) Arranging in-service training on health education methods and techniques.
(e) Research and evaluation of health education methods.

3 Health professionals Doctors, nurses, dentists, dietitians and paramedical staff are in a position to present health facts based on expert knowledge of the factors influencing health. Patterns of disease, methods of health care and prevention of ill-health constantly change, and there is a corresponding need in the professionals themselves for ongoing education and up-dating.

4 Other professional staff Many other professional workers have dealings with parents and children—teachers, nursery nurses, social workers and educational psychologists. These are people who have not usually received a medical or nursing training, but do have a knowledge of some of the important aspects of health promotion and are in a position to influence others.

5 Parents and other adults All parents are health educators for their children (although they may not regard themselves as such), by reason of the care they give, the environment they provide in the home, the inculcation of health habits and the examples they set. Parents themselves need to be aware of the extent of their direct and indirect influence, and to feel confident that they can help their child to value health. Although parents are the people most intimately and constantly in contact with the child, other adults in the child's expanding world also influence health attitudes, particularly those who are held in respect or esteem. It is important that all adults realise that their words and example affect children's views of what is desirable practice.

6 Children are usually regarded as the recipients rather than the promoters of health education. Nevertheless the health habits and persuasion of friends and older children may be a powerful health educational influence—for example, in smoking or not smoking. Some health education programmes in schools have been so effective in their impact that the children have acted as health educators for their parents in passing on information and suggesting ways in which they, the parents, might improve their own health and home environment.

7 Voluntary associations and societies Many societies produce educational leaflets and arrange courses and meetings on health topics.

8 The media The press, radio and television have great potential for health education, both directly through specific articles and programmes, and indirectly by incorporation of health education topics into popular series. Parents and children should be encouraged to develop a critical attitude to advertising which, understandably, presents the desirable aspects of a product in terms of consumer appeal, and omits or dilutes reference to factors which may adversely affect health.

9 The law At times, the law acts indirectly as a health educator by focusing attention on health topics such as the illegality of tobacco sales to children under 16 and the wearing of safety belts and crash helmets.

Health educators

1 The Health Education Council
2 Health education officer and staff
3 Health professionals—doctors, nurses, dentists and para-medical staff
4 Other professionals—teachers, social workers, nursery nurses and psychologists
5 Parents and other adults
6 Children
7 Voluntary societies
8 The media
9 The law

Methods of health education

There are many ways of providing health education, and choice is made of the methods most suited to the recipients in their particular situations.

1 Individual health education One-to-one health education takes place all the time when doctors, nurses, health visitors and midwives, meet patients and discuss health matters with them. The relationship between them is all-important; patients will listen to someone they know and trust, who they feel appreciates their circumstances and who speaks to them at their level of understanding.

2 Formal groups Health education may take the form of talks to groups of people such as mother and toddler groups or parent teacher associations. Such sessions need careful preparation on the part of the leaders and afford the opportunity for discussion and questions.

3 Technical aids These include booklets, leaflets, posters, tapes, slides and films, all of which are very valuable in reinforcing other methods of education, but should be chosen with care and used with discrimination. Their use should take into account:

(a) The wording of the text, so that it is easily understood and is capable of correct interpretation.

(b) The ability to read English or other languages—cartoons and clear illustrations are helpful in such circumstances.

(c) The ability to understand the spoken word. Tapes, captions and film commentary in the relevant mother-tongue should also be available.

4 Lectures and courses The Open University, adult and continuing education departments, Workers Education Association, voluntary organisations, paediatric departments and community health services provide a variety of lectures and courses on different health education topics, particularly aspects of parenthood, child care and development.

5 Campaigns A campaign supplements ongoing health education and takes place within a limited period of time, during which all forms of health education methods and material are concentrated on the one topic, such as 'Safety for Children', so that their combined impact on the public or selected groups will have maximum effect. Campaigns need careful planning to select the appropriate timing, co-ordinate methods of approach, ensure that health facilities are adequate to meet any increased demand as a result of the publicity, and to evaluate their effectiveness.

6 Indirect health education Financial inducement may act indirectly as a method of health education. The provision of free prescriptions and dental treatment for expectant mothers and children under the age of 16, and of free milk and vitamins when family income is low, emphasises the importance placed on medical and dental care and adequate diet.

Methods of health education

1 One-to-one communication
2 Group talks and discussion
3 Technical aids
4 Lectures and courses
5 Campaigns
6 Financial inducement

Stages in health education

Health education is an ongoing process throughout life; different age groups, or people in particular circumstances, have varying health needs at different times. Health education of parents helps good health practices and attitudes to develop in their family; children in turn are the parents of the future (Fig. 8.1). Within this health education cycle, the ante-natal period can be regarded as an arbitrary starting point, although it is hoped that, increasingly, young people will have been prepared for parenthood before pregnancy is contemplated, as health at the time of conception and the acceptance of responsibility for a child's well-being are very important.

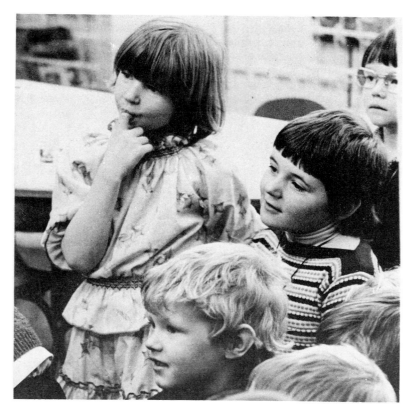

Fig. 8.1 Parents of tomorrow. *Colin New*

Health education in the ante-natal period

The ante-natal period is in many ways a time of good receptivity to health education, as the concern of the great majority of expectant parents is centred on the happy outcome of pregnancy and a desire to do everything possible to ensure the health of the baby. Both parents should be included in such educational programmes. In this period, health education takes place:

1   During routine ante-natal supervision by doctor and midwife, and through early contact of the family with the health visitor.
2   In classes held in the maternity unit or community clinic conducted by the midwife and health visitor, sometimes with the help of the physiotherapist and dietitian.

Health education is most effective when started early in the ante-natal period, and its content should include:

1   Simple explanation of the physiological changes taking place during the pregnancy, the purpose of screening procedures and of the different stages of labour. Relaxation exercises designed to help the efficient working of muscles during labour are included, and some idea is given of the various methods by which delivery can be made as easy and enjoyable as possible.

2   Explanation of ways in which the mother particularly can contribute to the well-being of the developing baby. This will include discussion on:

(a)   *Diet*: the needs of mother and fetus for adequate protein, minerals and vitamins.
(b)   *Smoking*, which is known to affect adversely the growth of the baby, both in utero and for some time after birth. Every effort should be made to encourage the expectant mother not only to stop smoking ante-natally but also to avoid resumption after delivery. Practical suggestions should be given about ways in which the habit can be broken with referral to an anti-smoking clinic if desired.
(c)   *Drugs*: in recent years, emphasis has been given to the possibly harmful effect of drugs, particularly if taken in the early months of pregnancy when the development of the fetus is at its most rapid stage. Advice is given to follow prescribed treatment only.

3   Information about the services and benefits available for expectant and nursing mothers, including:

(a)   *Pregnant women at work*: expectant mothers who are still working should know that they are legally entitled to paid time-off to attend an ante-natal clinic.
(b)   *Qualification for the maternity benefits*: the maternity grant is a single payment in respect of each baby and is not dependent on any insurance contribution having been paid by either the woman or her husband. The maternity allowance is a weekly benefit payable for up to 18 weeks, and dependent on the number of full-rate contributions paid by the woman herself. Full details of individual entitlement are obtainable from social security offices.
(c)   Free prescriptions and dental care.
(d)   Free milk and vitamins where family income is low.

4 Preparation for the changes in family life which pregnancy and the new baby introduce:

(a) The husband's role during pregnancy and after delivery. The traditional pattern wherein child-rearing is the almost exclusive role of the mother has long since past, and the importance of the father in the child's care and development is accepted.
(b) The effect of the new baby on other children in the family.
(c) Family planning.

5 The needs of babies and young children. Although the main focus of concentration for parents is usually the actual delivery, it is important to introduce the subject of child care during the ante-natal period. Parents can be helped to understand the baby's need for the close, intimate and loving relationships, and to realise the demands which are going to be made of them. Physical aspects of child care are also discussed—layette, bathing, warmth and type and frequency of feeding.

Infant feeding

A choice of two ways of feeding the baby—breast or bottle—is open to the mother. Health education is directed towards helping her make the wisest decision for her baby. Information is needed about the two methods, reasons for considering breast-feeding to be advantageous, and an awareness on the part of the midwife, health visitor and doctor of the various factors which influence the mother's decision one way or another.

Breast-feeding Although it is now possible for manufacturers to modify cows' milk so that in many ways it closely resembles human milk, breast-feeding is still considered to be the best method.

Advantages of breast milk This information can be given in simple terms to the mother:

1 It comes ready made-up in the right proportions, at the correct temperature, and its composition adapts to the baby's changing requirements.
2 Breast milk is less likely to lead to overweight babies.
3 It reduces the risk of hypocalcaemia and convulsions in otherwise healthy neo-nates.
4 Breast milk contains protective substances against infection which have not, as yet, been successfully incorporated into artificial feeds. Breast-feeding for even three to four weeks will help to protect the baby.
5 The risk of allergy is lessened.

6   There is very close contact between mother and baby during breast-feeding, which is satisfying for them both.
7   It has advantages for the mother:
    (a)   Ease of preparation.
    (b)   It helps to restore her figure in using up superficial fat.
    (c)   There may be some degree of protection against breast cancer.

Advantages of breast-feeding

1   Correct composition and temperature
2   Less likely to cause overweight babies
3   Reduces risk of hypocalcaemia
4   Protects against infection
5   Reduces risk of allergy
6   Encourages mother-baby relationship
7   Bonuses for the mother

Factors influencing breast-feeding   Health education to encourage mothers to breast-feed takes account of the many factors which influence its success or otherwise. Some of the more important influences include:

1   *Desire* on the part of the mother. The midwife and health visitor can give a great deal of encouragement by discussing with both parents the advantages of breast-feeding from the earliest weeks of pregnancy. Health education in schools, for both girls and boys, helps to foster positive attitudes towards natural feeding.

2   *Preparation*, which should begin in the ante-natal period with examination of the breasts and advice about their care in preparation for feeding.

3   *Expert help* from medical and nursing staff who are convinced of the advantages of breast-feeding, have practical knowledge about techniques, can explain them to the mother and have time and patience to assist her.

4   *Support at home* from the midwife and health visitor working in co-ordination to give continuous and consistent help and advice, and to maintain the confidence of the mother in her ability to breast-feed. Contact with other nursing mothers is often helpful, and bodies such as the Natural Childbirth Trust and the La Lèche League provide breast-feeding counsellors.

5   *The general climate* of opinion about breast-feeding which may profoundly influence a mother's decision; this is not only shown in

open comment, but is reflected more subtly in the general facilities (or lack of them) afforded to mothers who wish to feed their baby during shopping or on a journey.

Promotion of breast-feeding needs:

1 Desire on the part of the mother
2 Preparation in the ante-natal period
3 Support from professionals, family and society
4 Help in its establishment after birth
5 Help in its maintenance on return home

Artificial feeding Some mothers are reluctant or unable to breast-feed. It is important that in the general enthusiasm for breast-feeding they are not made to feel guilty, inadequate, or that their baby is getting second best. Mothers electing to bottle-feed need advice on:

1 *Choice*: there are many different varieties of modified baby milks, and there is little essential difference between them. Unmodified cows' milk ('doorstep' milk) is not recommended for babies in the early months of life because its composition in the crude form is so different from human milk that ordinary household methods are inadequate to modify it sufficiently to make it a satisfactory feed.
2 *Making up the feed* strictly according to the manufacturers' instructions so as to avoid the risk of over-concentration. Cooled boiled water can be offered twice a day in-between feeds.
3 *Sterilisation of equipment* by boiling or chemical methods.
4 *Importance of close contact* between mother and baby during feeding time, similar to that achieved during breast-feeding.

Supplements It is recommended that both breast- and bottle-fed babies are given extra vitamins. Human milk contains little or no Vitamin D; modified milks are fortified with this vitamin, but additional amounts in the prescribed dosage can be given. A combined preparation containing Vitamins A, D and C is provided by the Government at a low cost (free in the case of low income families) and is available from child health clinics.

Breast milk contains very little iron, but full-term babies usually have iron stores sufficient for their needs in the first 3–4 months of life. Some modified milk products are fortified with iron.

Weaning Some general advice about weaning is necessary during the period of full breast- or bottle-feeding. It is now agreed that the introduction of any food other than milk and vitamins should be unnecessary before the age of 4–6 months. There is no evidence that solid food given before this age is advantageous; indeed, it may introduce certain risks. For instance, the amount of salt in some weaning foods would place too much strain on the kidneys; also, the early introduction of gluten-containing cereals may predispose the early development of coeliac disease in a child who is sensitive to gluten. The use of rice, rather than wheat cereal, in the early weaning diet is recommended for all babies.

As the time for weaning approaches, discussion will include:

1   The purpose of weaning as a means of introducing the baby to a wide range of foods with different tastes, smells and textures which will meet the increasing needs of growth. By the age of six months, iron-containing foods such as eggs, green vegetables and liver are necessary. Weaning also encourages the baby to chew and bite, and in the use of a spoon and cup.
2   The need for weaning to be a gradual process, the duration of which varies from child to child.
3   Recognition of the individuality of each child, who will have his own initial reactions to change and may need introduction, interval, and re-introduction before accepting a new kind of feed.

Ante-natal health education includes:

1   Information about the changes during pregnancy and the stages of labour
2   The mother's contribution—diet, smoking and avoidance of drugs
3   Financial help and health care
4   Changes in family life
5   The needs of babies and young children

Health education in the early years

Health education in the early years of a child's life is directed towards helping parents understand the needs of young children and encouraging active participation in care so that they develop increasing confidence and gain much enjoyment from their family. Particularly with a first baby, or when supportive care from the extended family is not available, the midwife and health visitor, clinic doctor and general practitioner all have important parts to play in individual and group health education.

Topics on which health education is focused include:

1 *Relationships within the family*: the child's needs for love and security and the consistent framework of balanced discipline within the home.
2 *The developmental stages of childhood* (Chapter 6) with emphasis on the individuality of each child and ways in which his progress can be encouraged by new experience, toys, books and language.
3 *Infant feeding* and later diet.
4 *Safety in the home*: the visits of the health visitor provide good opportunities for assessing standards of home safety and the discussion of aspects of risk (Chapter 3).
5 *Protection against communicable disease*: how this can be achieved, the facilities available and discussion of doubts (Chapter 2).
6 *The use of available services*: where they are, what they provide and how to obtain them. This is particularly important for parents who have a child with a handicap or other special needs (Chapter 10 and Chapter 11).
7 *Dental health.*
8 *Preparation for specific events in a child's life*:

   (a) Going into hospital (Chapter 9)
   (b) The arrival of a new baby
   (c) Starting school.

Dental health education

Dental caries is one of the largest health problems of the present day, but because its effects are not life-threatening its prevention is often not regarded with the concern it deserves. Dental health education is appropriate in the ante-natal period not only for the expectant mother herself, but also to help lay down the foundations for strong teeth in the child by ensuring a diet adequate in calcium and Vitamin D. In childhood, education begins with helping the parents, and later the children themselves, to understand ways in which dental caries develops and what can be done to prevent it.

Dental caries results from erosion of the tooth by acid formed from sugar metabolism and bacteria, both of which are enclosed on the surface of the tooth by a film known as 'plaque'. The formation of plaque is encouraged by sweets and sugary foods, especially if given as snacks in-between meals. A particularly harmful practice is that of giving young babies sugar-containing fruit juices in a dinky feeder, or a dummy dipped in sugar or honey. If young children are started on healthy dietary habits these are easier to maintain into later childhood, especially if reinforced by education in dental health during their school years.

The first tooth usually appears between six and nine months of age, and tooth-brushing to remove any plaque should be encouraged from the start. Regular dental checks should begin early, regardless of whether there is any obvious indication of trouble. This accustoms the young child to the dentist and gives an opportunity for the dentist to discuss dental care with the mother.

The addition of carefully calculated small amounts of fluoride to drinking water is known to prevent dental decay by increasing the resistance of the tooth to acid. Although fluoridation of the water supply is one of the Government's health priorities, it has not yet been adopted in all health districts. Parents and children can be helped to appreciate the preventive value of fluoride and encourage the support of this measure. Where the water supply is deficient in fluoride, it can be taken by mouth in the form of tablets or drops. Fluoride solutions can also be applied to the teeth by a dentist; fluoride toothpaste also helps.

Prevention of dental decay

1 Avoiding sweets and sugary foods and drinks
2 Regular brushing of teeth
3 Regular dental checks
4 Fluoridation of water

The arrival of a new baby

A new baby in the family can demand quite a degree of adjustment on the part of a small child, particularly if he has, so far, been the only one. Wise preparation can help a great deal to smooth the way and prevent a child's natural feeling of some displeasure becoming a more difficult and lasting problem. The midwife and health visitor are in a position to help the parents in their approach.

An appropriate time to begin to prepare a child for the event is when the pregnancy becomes visible and preparations for the new baby are being made. It affords a good opportunity for early, simple health education on reproduction.

The mother will probably be delivered in hospital, and an explanation should be given to the child, with reassurance that she will soon be home again and that he will be looked after in her absence. The child needs to feel that he is still loved and wanted, even though there is a new brother or sister. He should be shown this in tangible terms, particularly by the mother making time to talk and play with him on his own.

Acceptance of the new baby into the child's family circle is helped by encouraging him to participate in care of the new baby. The parents need a sympathetic understanding of signs of insecurity and jealousy, such as temper outbursts, secondary enuresis and reversion to baby talk.

A new sibling

1 Preparation of the child during pregnancy
2 Reassurance of parental care and love
3 Participation in care of the baby
4 Recognition of signs of insecurity

Starting School

School entry is a feature in every child's life and the transition from a day spent largely at home to one of several hours away may be made simpler and more enjoyable by the health visitor discussing aspects of change with the parents.

Preparation of the child   Parents are encouraged to present school as an enjoyable experience. Make-believe play and illustrated story books can be used, and television programmes have been produced which look at this important milestone through a child's eyes. A preliminary visit to school is an opportunity to give the child a visual picture, to meet the head-teacher and know something about the programme of the school day and the degree of independence expected.

Diet   The contact of the health visitor in the early years will have familiarised the mother with the essentials of a healthy diet, but two points are valuable to mention:

1 *Breakfast*: the importance of breakfast is stressed in that it prevents tiredness, irritability and inability to concentrate.
2 *School meals*: mothers may be concerned about the child on a special diet or who dislikes unfamiliar food, has particular food fads, is a slow eater or a small eater. The health visitor, with her links with the school health service, can advise the mother about the flexibility within the school meals service.

Sleep   The amount of sleep needed varies from child to child, and the general aim is to try to achieve regular hours with consistency during term time. Bed-time should be recognised as a time when the day's experiences are often talked about and, therefore, should not be rushed.

Safety   The safety of children to and from school is a matter of concern. The child should know who is meeting him after school and, as far as is feasible for the child's age, an understanding of road drill should be assured, and the inadvisability of accepting lifts from strangers discussed.

Reaction to change Children react in different ways to the change of pattern in their day; the majority adapt easily to school life, particularly if they have had some previous experience in nursery school, day nursery or playgroup. There may, in some children, be temporary reactions for which parents should be prepared and helped to understand their significance:

1   Fatigue is common initially, especially after a whole day at school, but excessive activity may characterise other children.
2   Regression to immature behaviour at home can be a valuable safety valve if the demands which school makes for mature control are imposing a strain.
3   Enuresis may be a temporary reaction to change, or may be associated with some specific anxiety.
4   Physical symptoms such as abdominal pain, nausea and headache as school-time approaches are very real to the child.

The school health service The purpose of this service should be explained to the mother—what it offers, who the staff are, the pattern of surveillance and the desirability of the mother being present at the first medical examination to help the staff, reassure the child and discuss her child's progress.

Preparation for school

1   A pleasurable prospect for the child
2   Diet
3   Sleep
4   Safety
5   Recognition of signs of reaction to change
6   The school health service

Health education in the early years

1   Relationships within the family; the child's needs for love and security
2   Child development
3   Infant feeding and later diet
4   Home safety
5   Immunisation
6   The use of available services
7   Dental health
8   Preparation for special events; the arrival of a new baby and starting school

Health education for ethnic minority groups

The term 'ethnic minority' includes people of many different races and characteristics who have settled in this country; of the non-European groups those of West Indian and Asian origin are most numerous. It is essential for anyone undertaking health education to have a knowledge of the influential cultures, religions and customs, and to combine this with a sensitive and imaginative approach so that, where possible, health problems can be resolved in a way that is acceptable to educator and recipient.

Prevention of illness

Sickle cell anaemia is an inherited condition occurring in some West Indians, Africans and Asians, but not in people of English origin. An abnormal form of haemoglobin (HbS) can cause distortion of the red blood cells into a characteristic sickle shape, making them more liable to disintegrate, clump together and block small blood vessels. In the first year of life, this condition causes anaemic crisis, which may underlie respiratory or generalised infection; older children have episodes of severe abdominal and bone pain. Laboratory tests can identify HbS as early as the pre-natal and neo-natal periods. New methods of treatment are being developed. People at risk because of their race need information about sickle cell anaemia and facilities for diagnosis and genetic counselling.

Differences in the environment between this country and the country of origin indicate the need for preventive health measures. Lack of sunlight, low dietary intake of Vitamin D and dark skins combine to make rickets more prevalent than amongst white children (Chapter 5).

Advice on home safety and removal of old paint, possibly containing lead, helps to reduce the risk of accidents and ill-health arising from poor housing conditions and overcrowding (Chapter 1).

Many ethnic minority mothers followed the example of English women in the 1960s and early 1970s by electing to bottle-feed rather than breast-feed their babies. The community midwife and health visitor now spend considerable time in encouraging breast-feeding or, if this is not possible, demonstrate safe bottle-feeding procedures, making sure that instructions on constitution of feeds and sterilisation of equipment are understood.

Language difficulties

Attempts are being made in a variety of ways to solve difficulties of communication arising out of the inability to speak and read the English language. These include:

1   The use of interpreters who should have some training to familiarise themselves with health terms.
2   Translation of the written and spoken word into the mother-tongue, in leaflets, posters, tapes, and radio and television programmes.
3   English language classes originated by the education department for parents and children.
4   Home tuition for women in the use of the English language, which includes phrases most likely to be useful in hospitals or clinics.
5   Employment of more professional workers of the same ethnic group who would be able to communicate in language and thought.

Through these methods, it is hoped to help non-English speaking people to explain their health worries and queries, understand information, medical advice and procedures in hospitals and clinics, and to lead to a better utilisation of services.

Family life

Patterns of family life and child care differ from those commonly accepted in this country and a flexible approach enables services to meet the needs.

The health visitor, through her home visiting, helps to overcome the difficulty of initial reluctance to use the services. She has a particular concern for the isolation of some Asian women who are closely confined to the home and have very little contact with people other than family and women friends. She gradually encourages them to attend the child health clinic and use family planning facilities; the domiciliary service is particularly valuable.

Many West Indian and Asian mothers do not sufficiently appreciate the need for stimulation of children through toys, books and play, particularly outdoor play. The health visitor or home tutor can explain their importance and encourage the family to participate in play schemes for mother and child, playgroups and nursery classes.

Inter-marriage in some groups is common, resulting in an increase of inherited disorders. This, combined with the desire for a healthy male child, can at times make effective genetic counselling and contraceptive advice extremely difficult.

Tradition and religion

These important cultural elements must be appreciated:

1   Asian men are leaders of opinion and, through them, information and advice are transmitted to the women. Success in health education often depends largely on the initial approach to husbands or religious leaders.

2 Some dietary regimes are very restricted by religious taboos, leading to a risk of anaemia and difficulties when special diets are needed. Hospital dietitians and school meals staff are generally aware of the problem and try to provide meals which are acceptable.
3 Medical practices customary in the country of origin may persist in folk remedies and traditional 'cures' being sought before approaching the health services. The sale of dangerous remedies is banned, but health education on alternative care is a gradual process.
4 Traditional cosmetics, such as 'surma' used by children as well as adults, contain appreciable amounts of lead and their regular use can cause high lead levels in the blood.
5 Conflict may arise when parents insist on traditional behaviour in adolescent girls, who envy the relative freedom of their English friends.

Health education for ethnic minority groups

1 Appreciation of cultural patterns
2 Specific health problems
3 Help with language difficulties
4 Differences in family life
5 Tradition and religion

Health education in the school years

Health education in the first few years is mainly instilled through parental attitudes and example. When the child begins school life, education for health is a joint responsibility of parents and teachers, and there is a need for mutual consistency and reinforcement in the approach (Fig. 8.2). The aim of health education during school years is:

1 To give children information about how their body works and on health matters appropriate to their age.
2 To encourage thought and questioning.
3 To help them clarify their attitudes and values about themselves and other people.
4 To encourage them to discuss choices and make decisions.

Health education needs to be a continuous process throughout school life and its planning is best undertaken by the school teaching and counselling staff, together with the health service staff involved in the life of the school (Fig. 8.3). Its content will include:

1 Concepts of growth and physical development—the part played by diet, hygiene, dental health, exercise, smoking, alcohol and accidents.

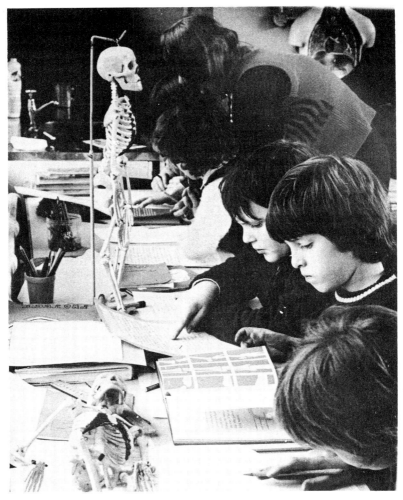

Fig. 8.2 Learning about health. *Colin New*

2　The emotional and social needs of children.
3　Sexual growth and development within the framework of family and
　　wider relationships.

There is a place for a variety of teaching methods (Fig. 8.4) and people
such as the doctor, school nurse, health visitor and marriage guidance
counsellor assist in the introduction of topics needing specialised
knowledge and approach. Surveillance procedures, medical examinations and counselling sessions with the school doctor and nurse can be
used as opportunities for health education.

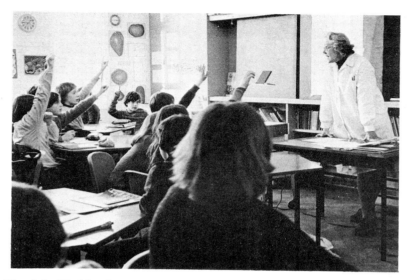

Fig. 8.3 Health education in school—participation of school health staff.
Colin New

Health education in school years

1 A joint responsibility of parents and school
2 Planned and taught by teaching and health staff
3 Helps children understand how their bodies work and to value health
4 Encourages thought and discussion about topics such as:
   Personal relationships
   Preparation for parenthood
   Smoking, alcohol and drugs

Important areas in health education which become increasingly relevant as adolescence and adulthood approach are:
1 Sex education
2 Education for parenthood
3 Social influences such as smoking, alcohol and drugs

Sex education

In the early years, a child absorbs from his parents ideas about and attitudes towards himself as a person, his body and the way it functions.

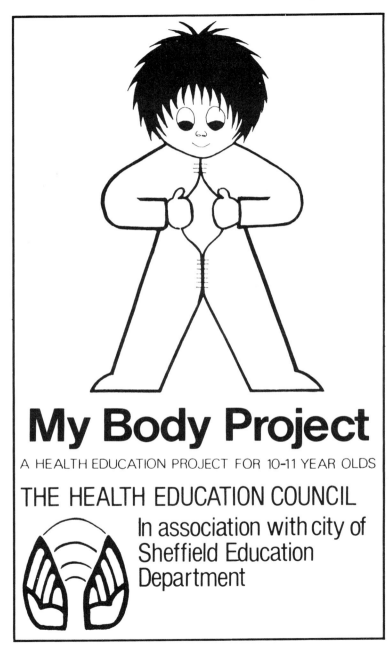

Fig. 8.4   'My Body', a health education project (see Appendix)

The patterns of relationships within family life, simple truthful explanations and answers to questions (aided by well-written and illustrated books) and the use of opportunities such as the mother's pregnancy, all help to prepare the young child for continuing education within the school. Sex education in schools should be planned with care and sensitivity and should aim to integrate biological information into the broader framework of relationships and responsibility, leading on to the subject of planned parenthood. The programme spans a number of years, during which different aspects and concepts are introduced at appropriate ages. Sex education includes:

1 Information on the anatomy and physiology of sexual development, its normal variations and relation to human reproduction. As the onset of puberty in many children today occurs in their primary school years, it is important that menstruation with its associated emotional and social aspects is discussed during this time.

2 Discussion of sexual relationships within the context of human behaviour. This part of sex education involves the discussion of principles and values, stresses the aspects of care, consideration and concern for others, and helps children develop the ability to envisage the consequences of their decisions and actions in relation to themselves and others.

3 Information about family planning and contraceptive measures. It is an accepted fact today that by the time children leave school many will have had some kind of sexual experience and some will have exposed themselves to the risk of an unplanned pregnancy. In addition to the biological and behavioural aspects of sex education, the importance of family planning needs emphasis, with simple general explanation of the various methods of contraception and ways of obtaining advice (Chapter 1).

4 Information about sexually-transmitted disease. Many children have heard about these conditions and want clear information about them; some may be at risk because of their promiscuous habits.

Components of sex education

1 The anatomy and physiology of human sexual development and reproduction
2 Discussion of relationships and responsibility
3 Family planning and contraceptive measures
4 Sexually-transmitted diseases

Sexually-transmitted diseases This term covers a variety of disorders, grouped together because of their common mode of transmission i.e. sexual intercourse. They include syphilis, gonorrhoea and other infections caused by bacteria, viruses, protozoa and parasites.

Syphilis

Organism: A spirochaete—*Treponema pallidum*

Transmission: From person to person by direct sexual contact. The spirochaete can also pass through the placental barrier and infect a fetus *in utero*

Incubation period: 10 days to 12 weeks, commonly about 21 days

Clinical signs: Three stages of syphilis, with varying lengths of duration, are described:

1 Primary syphilis shows as a painless sore (chancre) on the penis, the labia or within the vagina where it may not be seen. The sore clears up spontaneously, but the infecting organisms have passed into the blood stream.
2 Secondary syphilis appears within 6–12 weeks as skin rashes, mouth ulcers, enlargement of the lymph glands and fever.
3 Tertiary syphilis develops after an interval of years and can cause damage to almost every system of the body. Syphilis is diagnosed by identifying the spirochaete in smears from the primary sore, and by blood tests which give a positive reaction in the secondary and tertiary stages.
4 Congenital syphilis in a baby infected from the mother during pregnancy can cause still-birth, prematurity, neonatal death, and later handicaps such as blindness and deafness. Diagnosis and treatment in the ante-natal period have made this form of syphilis rare.

Treatment: Syphilis responds to treatment with penicillin, but damage to organs in the later stages is irreversible. No lasting immunity is conferred by one attack. Diagnosis and treatment are usually carried out in special clinics.

Gonorrhoea

Organism: A diplococcus—the gonococcus

Transmission: Direct sexual contact

Incubation period: 3–6 days

Clinical signs: Gonorrhoea causes a persistent, irritating discharge from the penis or vagina, with pain on micturition, but in women may often be symptomless. Later effects of gonococcal infection include arthritis and sterility due to epididymitis in the male and salpingitis with blockage of the fallopian tubes in the female. Gonococcal infection in the mother's vagina and cervix may reach the baby's eyes during delivery and cause ophthalmia neonatorum, a serious eye infection which can result in blindness.

Treatment: Penicillin and other antibiotics cure gonorrhoea in the early stages, but the gonococcus has developed increasing resistance to penicillin and large doses may be necessary to eradicate the infection. As with syphilis, an attack of gonorrhoea does not confer any future immunity.

Other sexually-transmitted diseases
These include:

1 Non-specific urethritis in men, vaginitis and cervicitis in women caused by the *Chlamydia trachomatis*.
2 Virus infections such as genital warts and genital herpes; incidence of the latter has increased greatly in the last 10 years.
3 Yeast infections and trichomoniasis, although both these are not necessarily the result of sexual intercourse.

Prevention and control   Ante-natal screening and prompt treatment of infection during pregnancy has done a great deal to eradicate congenital syphilis; the detection of gonorrhoea is less simple, as this requires routine taking and culture of cervical and vaginal smears and awareness of the possible significance of an unusual vaginal discharge.

Apart from the ante-natal screening, the main methods of prevention and control are in health education and contact tracing.

Health education

1 Gives information about the diseases, methods of transmission and signs arousing suspicion of infection. The wisdom of seeking advice, even in the absence of symptoms, if there has been any risk of infection should be stressed. It is important for young people to appreciate that sexually-transmitted diseases are not usually associated with a stable and permanent sexual relationship.
2 Gives details on how confidential advice, diagnosis and treatment can be obtained through special clinics.
3 Emphasises the need for early advice to be sought, not only for the safety of that particular person, but in order to enable contacts to be seen and examined.

Contact tracing

The District Health Authority is responsible for the tracing of contacts of people infected with a sexually-transmitted disease and a specialist health visitor or social worker is often employed for this purpose.

Sexually-transmitted diseases

1 Include syphilis and gonorrhoea
2 Are transmitted by direct sexual contact
3 Need early diagnosis and treatment
4 Control depends on ante-natal screening, health education and contact tracing

---

Education for parenthood

Responsibility for parenthood and the health of a future generation of children are health education topics which emerge from a consideration of human reproduction and personal relationships. There is a need for both boys and girls of all standards of academic ability to be included in specific programmes. The majority of older children are keenly interested in the prospect of their own future role as parents, and education for parenthood aims to inform them about the needs of young children and help them to understand the degree of commitment and responsibility required to fulfil these needs. Health education in this field includes:

1 Discussion on aspects of family life—a realistic as well as romantic appreciation of marriage and parenthood.
2 Information about the needs of the child for a good start in life—a planned and wanted conception, and co-operation on the part of parents in ante-natal care. Emphasis is given to factors influencing health and development and the value of a good environment, not only in the physical sense, but also in terms of the security based on love and affection.
3 Theoretical and practical teaching on aspects of child care such as diet, clothes, bathing, toys and play, together with time spent helping in playgroups, day nurseries or nursery classes.
4 The practical needs of family life—budgeting and household management, the demands of work and home, and the difficulties of unemployment.

Many schools are aware of the difficulties of finding time for such courses in a tight curriculum, but an increasing number are embarking on prescribed CSE courses in parentcraft or those arranged by organisations such as the National Association for Maternal and Child Welfare.

Education for parenthood

1 Relationships
2 Needs of children
3 Practical child care
4 Practical needs of family life

Social influence: smoking, alcohol and drugs

All these health education topics have multiple connotations which involve the physical, social and emotional aspects of life. Medical aspects should be discussed within the framework of personal relationships and individual and corporate responsibility.

Smoking and health   It is now accepted that regular smoking is a danger to health and that the habit, once started, is often very difficult to break. Health education programmes are likely to be most effective if started in the primary school and reinforced regularly during later school years. Children should be made aware of the facts about the effect on health of smoking:

1 Cigarette smoking greatly increases the risk of lung cancer, bronchitis and other respiratory disorders, and coronary thrombosis.
2 Smoking during pregnancy adversely affects the growth of the fetus and is also associated with increased perinatal mortality.
3 Smoking produces immediate respiratory disorders in children, even in those who smoke very little, such as coughs, colds, catarrh and shortness of breath after exercise.

The aim of health education is to help children relate the known facts about smoking and health to themselves, and produce positive inducements which will encourage non-smoking. Lung cancer is a long-term risk which they find difficult to appreciate but the advantages to a baby of a non-smoking mother are more likely to be influential, particularly amongst older girls. The relationship of smoking to respiratory disorders in their own age group can be presented in terms of better health, increased athletic potential and financial gain.

   Health education should take into account an appreciation of some of the factors influencing children to start and continue smoking:

1 Pressure from friends and the wish to follow the pattern of the peer group.
2 Family smoking habits in parents and, particularly, siblings.
3 The example of other adults such as teachers, youth club workers and popular public figures.
4 Television, particularly in programmes which present smoking as an indispensable attribute of manliness and feminine sophistication.
5 The ease, in spite of legal restrictions to the contrary, with which children under 16 years of age can buy cigarettes.

Health education at school is only a partial response to a broader need to provide children with an environment inwhich it is more desirable and easier not to smoke than to do so. A great deal has already been attempted by discouraging smoking on health premises and in some shops, but there is still a need for individual adults, parents in particular, to become more aware of the influence of their own attitudes and example.

Health education on smoking

1 Should start during primary school
2 Gives information about health risks
3 Encourages children to relate smoking to their own health
4 Examines reasons why children smoke
5 Includes parents and other adults

Alcohol   Drinking of alcohol has long been accepted in this country as a pleasurable social habit. The need for health education about alcohol arises because children do not always appreciate that its use may sometimes produce damaging effects to the individual and other people.

As with smoking, health education about alcohol should start during primary school years, when it can be most effectively used to help balanced, informed attitudes develop. Children should be made aware of the effects of the ingestion of alcohol:

1 Alcohol has a sedative rather than a stimulant effect on the brain, releasing inhibitions and slowing down reactions. Although small or moderate amounts produce a pleasurable effect, large amounts of alcohol can produce gross incoordination of movements, loss of the usual control over actions and emotions, and confusion. These consequences can not only endanger the individual, but can also affect the safety and happiness of others; alcohol is frequently a factor in road accidents, violence, hooliganism and vandalism.

2   Alcohol taken during pregnancy, either in relatively small regular amounts or large sporadic quantities, can result in growth retardation in the baby.

3   A proportion of people will become addicted to alcohol and the incidence of true alcoholism is increasing in the 25–30 years age group.

Some children may be introduced to alcohol at home, others at the instigation of friends, others start drinking because they see it presented as an acceptable part of adult life. The aim of health education is not necessarily to advocate total abstinence but to help children:

1   Understand the need for alcohol to be used wisely and in moderation.

2   Recognise that individuals vary in the degree to which they can tolerate alcohol, and that each one will have to recognise his own limits beyond which danger may lie.

3   Recognise early warning signals which signify loss of control, both in the immediate and distant future.

Parents, as well as the school, play a big part in health education on alcohol, and it may be helpful to involve them in health education programmes. Their own attitudes and drinking habits form part of the child's environment, and it is with their help that the child will become mature enough to resolve problems without recourse to the use of alcohol as a screen against difficulty.

Health education on alcohol

1   Should begin in primary school years
2   Gives information about the effects of taking alcohol
3   Helps children to develop a balanced attitude towards it
4   Involves parents

Drugs   It is difficult to assess the size of the problem where drug-taking is concerned because official statistics deal only with the numbers of registered addicts. It is probable that a great deal of experimentation with drugs takes place but stops well short of trouble. Nevertheless, there is a general concern, particularly amongst the parents of adolescents, about drug-taking of any kind, and the contribution which health education can make to prevention and control of drug abuse should be considered.

Health education recognises the complexity of the problem. The term 'drugs' covers a whole range of substances—sedatives, tranquilisers, stimulants, pain killers and, in an associated sense, alcohol, glue and certain solvents. It is not possible to describe here the individual properties of each different substance, but it can be said generally that:

1 Their indiscriminate use, particularly outside medical prescription and supervision, may result in side-effects which are undesirable, unexpected and unpredictable, and people vary a great deal in their reaction and tolerance to individual drugs.
2 They are capable of producing dependence which affects physical and mental health, social and emotional relationships. All the factors which result in some people, but not others, becoming dependent are not yet known.
3 Their abuse can affect others beyond the individual, such as the unborn child, members of the family and, through violence and crime, society in general.

Drugs are taken by young people for a variety of reasons—as an experiment, the result of pressure from the peer group, or to maintain wakefulness (e.g. during all-night parties); as a relief from boredom, or to enliven what is felt to be a drab life; because of personality problems such as extreme shyness, or as a relief from stress.

Drug abuse should be seen in the context of modern life, when sedatives and tranquilisers are widely prescribed, and recourse to pills or drink is often seen to be the first and quick answer to the relief of problems which might be resolved in more constructive ways.

The task of health education lies in three directions:

1 The risks of drug-taking can be explained to young people, aiming to achieve a balance between giving the facts and not provoking experiment or causing alarm. It should be presented not as an isolated topic, but as part of a general programme in which aspects of adolescent health and relationships and problem-solving are discussed, with opportunities for questions and exchange of opinions.
2 Parents also benefit from health education to help them with understanding adolescent struggles and conflicts and possible reasons underlying the need for drug-taking, particularly any factors of stress in personal or family life. They should be made aware of people who could help with counselling and advice (such as school pastoral staff, doctors, social workers and clergyman), of the recognition of signs indicative of a drug problem and agencies providing treatment.
3 As a long-term undertaking, more education of the public as a whole is desirable regarding the use of drugs, whether prescribed or self-purchased.

Health education on drugs

1 Recognises the complexity of the problem
2 Emphasises the risk of dependency and possible effects on other people
3 Examines reasons for drug-taking
4 Helps children to understand the risks
5 Includes education for parents and community

Health education and the future

Those responsible for health education are constantly presented with new challenges as some health problems are solved and others emerge.

Some aspects of life alter very quickly, and people today are faced with adjusting to changing situations and expectations. It seems that a big task for health education in the future is in the field of helping to maintain not only physical health but also mental and emotional well-being in the face of situations which could undermine self-esteem, such as unemployment.

Parents today are often faced with very difficult decisions arising out of dilemmas of choice in medical care—for instance, the recent debate about the efficacy and safety of whooping cough vaccine. Perhaps yet another field of health education is to help parents accept the challenge of choice and to be able to tolerate the anxiety that sometimes accompanies it.

A recurrent challenge is that of reaching those for whom health education would appear to be beneficial but who are not sufficiently motivated to take advantage of conventional methods. New lines of approach should always be considered, including the involvement of neighbourhood individuals who, though not primarily educators, could, after simple basic training, achieve a great deal through being accepted by the family because they come from the same background, have similar experiences and speak the same language.

Health education is an important part of the community health services. Its results are sometimes recognised immediately, but often may need a span of years in order to reveal their full effect. Perhaps as important a challenge as any to health education is that of evaluating its own achievements.

9
Services for Children

It is only within the last 100 years or so that the child has been generally accepted as an individual person in his own right with special needs to be met. The organisation of total care involves the integration of many medical and nursing skills, together with the expertise of workers in other disciplines, particularly social services and education.

Planning of local child health services is the responsibility of the district management team working within the broad policy framework laid down by the Department of Health. They are assisted by medical and nursing staff with special interest and responsibility in child health matters, and by special planning groups which include doctors, nurses and representatives of the local authority education and social services departments.

Present-day child health services offer a wide range of provisions, which include:

1 Prevention of ill-health and handicap, both immediately and for the future.
2 Support and advice for parents and others who may be involved in the care of the child, so that they may understand ways of promoting good health, how to recognise illness, and the appropriate action to be taken.
3 If and when illness does occur, prompt treatment and care of the ill child, whether at home or in hospital.

The community child health services

These services are mainly preventive in function, seeking through surveillance, immunisation, health education and counselling for children and parents, to promote good health both in the present and for the future. They work closely with other branches of the National Health Service, and the social services and education departments, in the co-ordinated care and support of ill or handicapped children who return to their homes in the community after diagnosis and treatment in hospital. The community services are concerned with the needs of the total child population, and try to ensure that as high a proportion as possible of all the children within the district benefit from the preventive services available. The birth notifications form the basis of a system which enables health records of all children to be compiled; when families move from district to district, transfer of information takes place. The use of computer systems is increasing and this facilitates the making of appointments for immunisation and surveillance procedures, and the follow-up of defaulters. Because the community services reach out to all children, it is possible to compile statistical data about standards of health, prevalence of handicapping conditions, use of services and evaluation of present and future needs.

The District Health Authority has a legal responsibility to give advice and support to the education and social services departments of the local authority, and this is undertaken by community medical and nursing staff. Community health services have historically evolved in association with the provision of health services to schools, and this remains one of their important functions, particularly in regard to children with disabilities likely to affect their capacity to learn. The community child health services include:

1 Child health clinics
2 School health service
3 Community health staff
4 Community dental service
5 Health education service

Child health clinics

The function of a child health clinic remains similar to that of the original ones established at the end of the 19th century—to follow the progress of a child until school entry and to give advice and support to the parents. Over the years their scope has broadened as more has become known about child health and development, and the original emphasis on physical health has extended to cover all aspects of health and development, particularly in the emotional field, and a wide range of social problems. The principal activities in a child health clinic are:

1 Surveillance of growth and physical, mental, social and emotional health (Chapters 4 to 6).
2 Recognition of medical conditions, acute or chronic, with referral for investigation or treatment.
3 Advice to parents on any health problem or difficulty in management they may wish to discuss—for example, feeding procedures, behaviour problems, sleep difficulties and immunisation.
4 Immunisation against diphtheria, whooping cough, tetanus, polio and measles.
5 Health education, both formal and informal. Mother and toddler groups are also held on clinic premises.
6 The sale of proprietary brands of infant foods and vitamin preparations at an economic price and the issue of free milk and vitamins for those entitled.

Access to the clinic should always be open, although special appointments can be made for some sessions. Attempts are made to site clinics at positions of maximum ease of access, so that ideally they can act as neighbourhood centres. When this is not possible, mobile clinics may be provided.

The clinics are usually staffed by a clinical medical officer and a health visitor. In some areas, consultant paediatricians also participate in clinic activities, either by undertaking a routine session or by holding a consultation clinic on the premises.

Child health clinic activities

1 Surveillance of health and development
2 Advice and support to parents
3 Immunisation
4 Health education
5 Sale of milk and vitamin preparations

The continuing need for child health clinics has been debated. Ideally, the family doctor is the person who should be responsible for the total health care of the child, including surveillance of development, immunisation and counselling of parents. He is the person who knows the child and the inter-relationships with the family, enabling him to detect early signs of illness and abnormality and thus being well-equipped to provide continuity of care in health and in sickness. An increasing number of general practitioners are becoming interested in the preventive aspects and hold 'well-child' clinics on their surgery premises. In some districts, the whole of the preventive pre-school child health services are already undertaken by a general practitioner himself or by a clinical medical officer working on behalf of the practice.

The school health service

The school health service is concerned with the health of school children, particularly in relation to their ability to benefit from education. Ideally, each school should have its 'named' doctor and nurse who would be regarded by teaching staff, parents, and children as part of the school. Functions of the school health service include:

1 Surveillance of children throughout school life (Chapter 7).
2 Hygiene inspections regarding cleanliness, head infestation and veruccas.
3 Immunisation programmes to boost previous primary protection

against diphtheria, tetanus and poliomyelitis, and to offer BCG and rubella immunisation.
4 The identification and management of children with specific difficulties. The school health service staff are involved in the placement of a child in a suitable type of school, in reviewing progress and giving advice on the medical aspect of disability in relation to educational needs. Doctors and nurses working with handicapped children, whether in special schools or, increasingly, in ordinary schools need a knowledge of the medical, educational and social aspects of handicap and to develop close links with consultants, teachers, social workers and therapists involved in other aspects of the child's educational life.
5 Special clinics. Although the majority of treatment facilities still remain with the general practitioner and hospital service, there are some health concerns (for instance obesity, enuresis and early behaviour problems) for which the school health service can offer special counselling clinics. The value is recognised of integrated audiology and ophthalmic services in which school health service and hospital staff both work.
6 Assisting with health education in schools, which includes planning of, and participation in, programmes not only for children but also for their parents and teachers, regarding the effects of medical, surgical or social conditions on the child's ability to learn.
7 Advice on specific health problems in relation to:
 (a) *Work.* Physical or mental handicap or chronic illness may restrict the type of work which some children will be able to undertake, whether it be a proposed full-time occupation or out-of-school-hours job. The school doctor is able to advise on this, and should have close links with the careers officer and the employment medical advisory service.
 (b) *Suitability for free milk.* The practice regarding free milk varies in different local authorities. Some education authorities provide no free milk, whilst others make it available on health grounds or if the child is attending special school.
 (c) *The need for special transport* to school.
 (d) *Special diets* which the school meals service may be asked to provide for children with, for example, coeliac disease or phenylketonuria.
8 General advice to the local education authority on medical matters which may have implications for the planning of educational services.
9 Liaison with workers in other disciplines who are also involved in the educational aspect of a child's life, particularly the teaching staff, educational psychologist, and the education welfare officer.
10 Participation in research projects.

The school health service activities

1 Surveillance of children throughout school life
2 Hygiene inspections
3 Immunisation programmes
4 Work with handicapped children
5 Special counselling clinics
6 Health education
7 Advice on specific health problems
8 Advice to education department on planning of services
9 Liaison with other professional workers
10 Participation in research

Community health staff

Clinical medical officers   These are doctors working in the pre-school clinics and school health service, undertaking surveillance, immunisation, health education advice and counselling. They should have:

1 Some experience in paediatrics.
2 A knowledge of child development and the special needs of handicapped children.
3 An awareness of social problems which might influence health, development, educational progress, and behaviour.

Some doctors have a special expertise in the field of audiology and handicap, working in close association with the assessment clinics. Others may develop particular interests such as the epidemiology of childhood illnesses, non-accidental injury, early behaviour problems, obesity and enuresis. The clinical medical officer's work is of a preventive and advisory nature; they do not generally prescribe treatment, but refer children to the family doctor or hospital. Good communication between doctors in all the services is essential to enable consistent advice to be given to the children and parents, and maximum help to teachers. There is an increasing amount of interchange between medical staff working in the community service, general practice and hospital.

Clinical medical officers

1 Undertake preventive health work in the pre-school clinic and the school health service.
2 Work closely with other professional medical and nursing staff, and with teachers.

The health visiting service The health visitor is a state registered nurse who has taken an approved course in obstetric nursing and a further year's training in development of the individual, sociology and preventive health, in a university or polytechnic. She has a responsibility for the family as a whole, and as well as a specific concern for the mother and child, is also involved with the needs of the elderly. The health visitor's work in the field of child health includes:

1 Establishing initial contact with the expectant parents during the ante-natal period which will develop into a continuing relationship after the baby is born. The health visitor participates jointly with the midwife in health education.

2 *Home visiting.* The initial visit to the new baby is usually made about the 10–11th day after birth. The community midwife may also be visiting during the first 28 days, and it is important for the health visitor to liaise with her so as to avoid conflicting advice being given. On her first visit the health visitor assesses the family scene and talks with the parents on matters such as baby care, feeding and immunisation; this visit includes the start of surveillance, which she will maintain until at least the time of school entry. Many health authorities have evolved programmes of visiting which ensure that every child is seen a minimum number of times during the early years of life and, at the same time, leave flexibility for increased frequency of visiting should the health visitor consider this necessary in the case of individual families.

3 *Identification of families with special needs.* In some instances the health visitor becomes aware of situations which call for extra visiting and, possibly, the arrangement of special help for the family. For instance:
    (a) The young, inexperienced mother without the support of extended family.
    (b) The child with a handicap.
    (c) Families where there is a risk of violence, particularly non-accidental injury to the child.
    (d) The socially deprived family where unemployment may be an additional factor.
    (e) Non-English speaking families.

The health visitor is aware of agencies offering specialised services and can put the parents in touch with them.

4 Sessions at the child health clinic or the general practitioner's surgery, where mothers know they may call to see the health visitor in-between home visits if they particularly wish to do so. In many clinics, mother and toddler groups are initiated by the health visitor, giving opportunities for mothers (particularly the socially

isolated) to meet together on an informal basis, and for health education to be given.

5   Health education, which is an important aspect of health visiting.

6   Visits to playgroups and day nurseries whose staff welcome advice on health matters and, in turn, afford the health visitor opportunities to observe the progress of the children and meet with the mothers.

7   Visiting in cases of some communicable illness. This formerly amounted to a large part of the work of health visitors, but with the decline in incidence of many communicable diseases, is now only a proportionally small section. The health visitor's contribution lies in general advice to parents and the tracing of contacts in cases of serious illnesses.

8   Liaison with hospital units. Many paediatric, maternity and assessment units have a health visitor who acts as a co-ordinator of hospital and community services and information. The liaison health visitor also arranges for the follow-up of clinic defaulters.

9   Links with voluntary bodies. Many voluntary agencies are able to give special forms of help to families and it is important that the health visitor is aware of the available provisions, and how they may be obtained.

10 Nominated health visitors are members of the district handicap team, various special planning groups concerned with child health services, and attend case conferences when a particular family situation is being discussed.

11 The nature of health visiting work and the close contact with children and families in the community invites participation in various research projects.

At the present time, many health visitors are 'attached' to general practice, being concerned with the patients of one or more general practitioners with whom they work in close conjunction, thus enabling better communication and a combined approach to family health care. Where primary health care teams operate, the health visitor is an important member. Other health visitors are responsible for all the families (whoever their general practitioner may be) living within a defined geographical area. This has the advantage that the health visitor is regarded as a familiar and easily approachable person within her 'patch', and families with no general practitioner are less likely to 'slip through the net'. In some areas, where general practitioners work within a well-defined radius, attachment and geographical patch system can be successfully superimposed, bringing together the advantages of both.

Perhaps the two features of the health visiting service that warrant special emphasis are that it is the only service which actively seeks out children rather than waiting for parents to find the service, and that it is the only reliable means by which the progress of virtually *all* young children can be followed-up.

The health visitor

1 Actively seeks out children and families, aiming to see every child on her caseload
2 Is concerned with preventive child health, and works closely with the general practitioner and clinic doctor
3 Visits the home regularly to observe the child's progress and identify special needs
4 Supports and advises parents on the care of their children
5 Is a health educator
6 Links up with the school health service, the paediatric units, and statutory and voluntary agencies

---

The community midwife In recent years, many more births are taking place in hospital and a home delivery is a comparatively rare event. Nevertheless, the community midwife has an important role to play in ante-natal and post-natal care, and in some instances is able to conduct the confinement in the hospital maternity unit. During the ante-natal period the community midwife assists the general practitioner in ante-natal supervision and provides health education, both in her discussions with individual women and in parentcraft classes. When the mother and baby return home after delivery, the community midwife is responsible for their care at least until the 10th day of the puerperium, and may in some instances continue to visit for the first 28 days of the baby's life. This is a most important period, when the midwife can be of immense help to the new mother in assisting her to adjust happily to the new situation and in establishing feeding practices, particularly if breast-feeding. She also advises on family planning. The community midwife and health visitor should work closely together, both in the ante-natal and post-natal periods.

The community midwife

1 Shares in ante-natal care
2 May conduct delivery in hospital
3 Gives care to the mother and new baby in the early post-natal period

The district nurse sometimes known as the *home nurse* (page 163).

The school nurse   Different health districts vary in the organisation of the school nursing service. In some, the health visitor is also the school nurse, although she may delegate some of her school duties to a qualified assistant. In others, the service is distinct from the health visiting service, albeit maintaining close links. The school nurse in this case is a state registered nurse, who may have had special experience in other branches of nursing such as sick children's, ophthalmic or ear, nose and throat nursing or psychiatric work. The Council for Education and Training of Health Visitors has recently approved a 12 weeks' course in school nursing, designed to cover aspects of child health and development in school-age children, and to set these in the educational context so as to give insight into the different ways in which nursing skills can be utilised as part of school health work.

The duties of a school nurse include assisting the school doctor in programmes of surveillance and immunisation sessions, carrying out measurements of growth and other screening procedures, and making hygiene inspections. Her main emphasis is on the preventive aspect of child health including health education, to which her frequent contact with the children can contribute a great deal. She is also a very valuable link with the child's home, carrying out special visits to ensure that advice and treatment are being followed, obtaining social data which would assist the school doctor, helping parents whose child is home on holiday from special residential schools, and linking up with educational welfare officers regarding absentees from school. Other grades of nursing staff may also be employed in some school health services, working closely with the school nurse in routine hygiene inspections and growth checks.

The role of the school nurse

1   Assisting the school doctor in surveillance
2   Advice and counselling in the school
3   Health education
4   Hygiene inspections
5   Home visits

Other staff such as dietitians, speech therapists and physiotherapists may divide their time between the school health service, hospital and domiciliary work. Speech therapists provide help for children, pre-school as well as school-age, who have speech and language difficulties, either singly or associated with other handicap. They, and the physiotherapists, are particularly involved in therapy of the handicapped.

The community dental service

This service is staffed by qualified dentists and dental hygiene assistants and provides preventive dentistry and free treatment where necessary for all pre-school and school-age children, and for women during pregnancy and for a year after delivery. It is recommended that each school should be visited annually for the dental inspection of children, following which parents are notified of any treatment recommended (such as filling, extraction, scaling or polishing) and are given the choice of the child attending the community dental clinic or a family dentist. The community dental service participates in dental health education, arranging programmes for clinics, schools and the general public. Much informal education on a one-to-one basis takes place during inspections or dental hygiene procedures.

The health education service

This service has an important role in preventive health and its activities are discussed in Chapter 8.

The primary care team

The primary care team includes the general practitioner, health visitor, district nurse, and sometimes the community midwife, school nurse and social worker (page 168). This group can, amongst its members, provide a wide range of care, including preventive measures and health education as well as the diagnosis, treatment and nursing care of ill patients. The team approach to care enables efficient use of time and expertise; improved communications lead to sharing information about the family as a whole.

The general practitioner

The 'family doctor' is usually the parents' first line of approach, particularly for ill children. An increasing number of general practitioners now undertake preventive aspects of health care for the child and family. Practitioners may work single-handed but often several work together in a group practice accommodated in a medical or health centre, which forms an ideal basis for the primary health care team. Within a group practice there may be opportunities for one member to develop a special interest in child health and undertake most of this work, particularly in the preventive field, on behalf of the others. Some general practitioners also work on a sessional basis in the child health clinics or the school health service. General practitioners undertake to give a 24-hour service, but during the night one member of the group may act on behalf of the others, or arrangements may be made through a deputising service. It is estimated that approximately 25 % of all consultations handled by general practitioners are concerned with children, and from 1981 the compulsory vocational training scheme includes a six months' paediatric course.

Despite arrangements for general practitioner cover, it is estimated that about 20 % of families are not registered with a general practitioner, and this leads to difficulties not only in the case of acute illness, but also in identifying families with children so that health visiting services can be arranged.

Many mothers are uncertain about the urgency of calling the doctor if they are worried about their child's health; they are afraid of appearing over-anxious and appreciate some guidance as to when immediate help is indicated.

The following guidelines can be given in order that medical advice should be sought as a matter of urgency in cases of:

1   Injuries (especially head injuries), poisoning (whether suspected or definite), burns and scalds unless very slight, and obvious or suspected fractures.

2   Convulsions which, in young children, are often associated with sudden high temperatures that mark the beginning of many childhood infections. A convulsion may also denote epilepsy or may be an early symptom of meningitis or encephalitis.

3   Respiratory symptoms such as croup, or a croupy cough, difficulty in breathing, cyanosis, or an asthmatic attack which is not responding to the usual prescribed measures.

4   Abdominal symptoms, such as unusual or severe abdominal pain, vomiting and diarrhoea (which can be dangerous in babies and young children as dehydration develops very quickly). Repeated vomiting and diarrhoea need urgent attention, particularly if the stools are watery, or if associated with abdominal pain or a high temperature.

5   Patterns of behaviour which are unusual to that child. Observant parents notice changes such as repeated refusal of feeds, loss of appetite or unusual drowsiness; persistent crying which is unusual in its duration, pitch, intensity or apparent association with pain, needs investigation.

6   Acute otitis media with symptoms of severe pain, pyrexia and later discharge from the ear.

7   A child not responding, within the period, to prescribed treatment or if his condition is getting worse.

Infections such as measles, chicken-pox and mumps are common in young children. When such infections are known to be prevalent in the community, the doctor should be contacted about a child developing characteristic symptoms, but not necessarily as a matter of extreme urgency unless the child's general condition is obviously giving rise for concern.

Parents consent to medical and dental treatment on behalf of their child. When the age of 16 is reached, a young person is able by law to consent to or refuse treatment without reference to his parents. When the parents refuse treatment for a child, a doctor may proceed if the child's life is considered to be in danger. The parent's decision regarding treatment can also be challenged in court by making the child a ward of court or through care proceedings initiated by the local authority social services department (Chapter 11).

The district nursing service

The district nurse is a member of the primary health care team, working both in the home and in the doctor's surgery, and also maintaining links with the hospital. She has had further training to enable her to cope with the different situations which may arise when nursing care in the home is needed. Most district nurses work in small teams which include a state registered nurse, a state enrolled nurse and a nursing auxiliary. The district nursing service is available for patients of all ages but the number of children needing this service is comparatively small. The district nurse would:

1 Help with the care of an ill child at home, particularly in assisting and advising the mother in meeting the child's needs.
2 Give post-operative nursing care, especially after short-stay surgery.
3 Help in the care of children with chronic conditions such as diabetes, acting as a link between hospital services and the home. She would attend the relevant hospital clinic and become known to the parents as a person who can give advice and support in any anxiety that may arise.

Although children form a relatively small proportion of the district nurse's work, it is possible that more paediatric nursing care could be developed, either by encouraging some specialisation within the service or by using paediatric nurses working both within the hospital and in the community, thus bringing their special expertise in the care of the sick child out into the child's home and ensuring continuity of care.

A wide range of nursing equipment for use in the home is available on loan from the health authorities.

The primary care team

1 General practitioner
2 Health visitor
3 District nurse and practice nurse

And sometimes:
4 Community midwife
5 School nurse
6 Social worker

Hospital services

Hospital services for children include facilities for investigation, diagnosis and treatment of illness or handicap, both on an out-patient and in-patient basis. These services are available in specially designated children's hospitals and in paediatric units within a general hospital. Regional and sub-regional centres are set up for the investigation and treatment of uncommon conditions needing specialised forms of treatment. Some children, particularly those with ENT or eye conditions may be admitted to beds which are in mainly adult units and concern has been expressed that their special needs as children are not being met. Whatever type of hospital, unit or ward children are in, it is essential that their overall medical and nursing care should be in the hands of doctors and nurses who have special knowledge of, and training and experience in, the needs and care of children in health and sickness.

Although hospital facilities are not considered strictly to be 'community' services, it is essential where children are concerned not to regard them as isolated institutions.

Accident and emergency departments

It is estimated that approximately one child in six attends a hospital casualty department each year, and it is in this area that the overlap with the community aspect of care is often seen so vividly. Some parents use the department as an alternative form of primary care, rather than seeking the advice of their family doctor, particularly when the child's condition and their anxiety become acute outside the conventional working hours. In other instances, complicated and difficult social problems are uncovered during the investigation of an apparently minor accident or illness. In such situations the liaison health visitor and medical social worker act as links with community staff. Accident and emergency departments provide information on substances commonly ingested by children and can be contacted by telephone for immediate advice in an emergency.

Child psychiatric services

Special services are needed for children with emotional difficulties such as anxiety and depression and with severe behaviour problems. In adolescence, true psychotic illness may emerge, although this is relatively uncommon. It has been estimated that 5–10 % of children have psychiatric disorders severe enough to be termed handicaps. The child psychiatric service is staffed by consultant child psychiatrists, clinical psychologists, social workers and nursing staff, and includes facilities for out-patient consultation and in-patient stay. The service is particularly orientated towards family as well as child therapy, recognising that home and social influences play a great part in psychiatric disorders. The child psychiatric service works closely with other professionals in the community who are providing either a specialist type of counselling and therapy, such as the educational psychologist, or who may constitute the first-line of approach by the parents, such as the general practitioner, clinical medical officer, health visitor, school nurse and social worker.

Hospital attendance

For a proportion of children hospital attendance, and maybe admission, are episodes in their life when links with home and community must be preserved if the child is to receive maximum benefit. Whenever possible, the child is seen on an out-patient basis but if admission is considered advisable, the stay is made as short as possible.

Day care units Some hospitals include a paediatric day care unit to which children can be admitted on a daily basis. Day care units are used for:
1 Investigations which do not need full in-patient stay.
2 Observation of, for instance, the child with feeding difficulties or the constantly crying child. The nursing staff and medical social worker may be able to discuss problems with the parent and offer helpful suggestions on management.
3 Surgical procedures suitable for day-care facilities.

Longer in-patient stay inevitably involves some separation of the child from his parents at a time when he is most in need of their reassuring presence. This can be extremely distressing, particularly if he is not old enough to understand explanations. The older child may have vivid fears about hospital or medical and surgical procedures. Whatever the age, certain steps can be taken to make the stay as pleasant and untraumatic as possible.

Preparation for hospital   Everyday life events, books, games and television programmes, if used positively and skilfully by parents and teachers, can introduce children to the existence and purpose of hospitals, doctors, nurses and ambulance men, without causing undue anxiety. When admission to hospital is planned in advance, there is the opportunity for parents to prepare the child more specifically by simple explanation of why he is going there, stressing the positive aspect of being made better. Questions are answered truthfully and some idea of hospital routine given; many paediatric units supply leaflets giving this information for parents. It is most important for the child to know that his parents will be able to visit him and that they will come to take him home as soon as possible. A favourite toy, book or cuddly article helps to preserve the links with home.

Hospital visiting   Ideally, mothers should be with their child (particularly the very young) throughout the period of hospital stay, although this is not always practicable. Visiting should be unrestricted so that parents have the opportunity to be with their child for as long a period as possible each day and provisions are often made for overnight stay. The nursing staff can help parents by explaining ward routine and ways in which they can participate in the care of their child. Some parents may have difficulty in reconciling the needs of their child in hospital with those of other young children at home. Transport to hospital may be expensive. The hospital medical social worker is available to discuss these situations and offer practical help and advice. Some paediatric units have introduced a scheme of 'ward grannies' who will visit children regularly when parents find it impossible to do so.

Play and education   Play for children is as important in the hospital day as in home life; not only is it a means of employing time pleasantly, but it enables the child to express feelings which he may not be able to articulate, such as fear, anger or resentment. Play workers may form part of the ward team and assist children in individual and group play. For the child of school-age, continuity of education is important, particularly if the stay is long or recurrent. The Local Education Authority has a responsibility to provide teaching facilities for any child of statutory school age who is expected to remain in hospital for more than two weeks or has recurrent admissions.

Aftermath of hospital stay   (Fig. 9.1) The continual reassuring presence of parents during hospitalisation does a great deal to foster the

Going to Hospital

I run on the road and
I got noct down and I
had to go to The hospital
and they put a bagndged it up and I
luct at the nails wot the babys
had swollowed and they had
swallowed a magn er and
I went home in my daddys
car and I laid on the
settee eeting sum
sweers

my mummy told me
that I had been in Hospital
4 A year and I
wos in A glas frame
I wos nearly dying
with the pneymonia
and at last I came
home brely and spackling
and my mummy luvd me

Fig. 9.1 *Going to Hospital* by Mark, aged 6

child's sense of security. Not only does this help him during the time in hospital, but it may also prevent or lessen traumatic emotional after-effects. Parents need to understand that there may be a period following return home before the child is able to incorporate satisfactorily his recent experience into his life, and that for a time there may be reversion to more infantile patterns of behaviour, such as unwillingness to leave his mother and bed-wetting.

Stay in hospital

1 Should be as short as possible
2 Needs preparation of the child
3 Unrestricted visiting by parents
4 Facilities for play and education
5 May sometimes give rise to temporary emotional upset after return home

---

The Community Health Council

This is a body set up in 1974 as part of the National Health Service, to represent the consumer where the provision and delivery of health services are concerned. The council provides information on services, investigates complaints and instigates surveys on the functioning and quality of health services. There is one council in each health district and members include representatives of the local authority and voluntary organisations, together with people appointed by the Regional Health Authority.

The social services department

This is a local authority department responsible, since 1971, for the care and welfare of people, including children, particularly where there are difficult home circumstances.

Social workers   The social services department employs social workers who work mainly in the community and are responsible for giving support, advice and help to families and their children who otherwise would not be able to cope with their personal or social problems or make good use of existing services. A community social worker may be a member of the primary care team, sharing knowledge of families and providing sustained counselling and support in difficult social circumstances. Medical social workers are based in hospital and deal with social problems encountered in families whose children are attending the hospital. They link up on the one hand with hospital medical and nursing staff and the liaison health visitor, and on the other hand with community care teams and social workers.

Short- and long-term care The department makes arrangements for the day care of children in local authority nurseries, and full-time care by fostering or in community homes or hostels. It has duties in the registration of private day nurseries and child-minders (Chapter 11), and in connection with private fostering and homes. It also acts as an adoption agency.

Special help Home helps and home makers are employed by the department to give assistance with housework or the care of children, in the case of the mother's illness or handicap, or where the parent's inability to cope with their children's care might otherwise result in family breakdown.

Family centres are provided, offering facilities for parents and children such as toy libraries and play sessions. Special help is also provided for the handicapped child and his family, such as adaptations to the home and equipment to help in daily living.

When circumstance demands, the social services department can apply for legal measures to protect children from physical, emotional or moral danger.

Social services department

1 A local authority department
2 Provides social workers
3 Makes arrangements for short- and long-term care
4 Acts as an adoption agency
5 Provides special help for handicapped and disadvantaged

The education department

The local authority education department, as its name implies, is responsible primarily for the provision of education for all children between the ages of 5 and 16 years or beyond. In recent years, much importance has been placed on facilities for education in nursery schools and classes for children under the age of five, particularly those living in deprived areas who might otherwise lack the stimulation and variety of experience needed for development. The education department recognises the inter-relationship of health and general well-being with the child's ability to benefit from education and, in addition to the department's close links with the health services, appoints staff who are particularly involved with the social and behavioural aspects of a child's life.

The school psychological service is part of the local authority education department and is staffed by educational psychologists who are teachers with an additional qualification in psychology. Educational psychologists give help to children whose school progress or behaviour is causing concern, and they are particularly involved in the assessment of educational needs of handicapped children. This service forms part of the network of services available for children with psychiatric disorders.

The education social work service also administered by the education department, is concerned with social problems in school children and their families. The education welfare officer may be involved in investigation of non-attendance at school, arrangements for the provision of school meals, clothing, transport, and in the referral of families to other agencies who could provide special help.

Child care assistants are usually qualified nursery nurses who assist the teaching staff in:
1 Nursery schools, with the general care and supervision of the young child.
2 Ordinary schools, where the feasibility of a handicapped child being educated there may depend on help being available for toilet routines.
3 Special schools, where many handicapped children may need assistance.
The child care assistant works very closely with the school nurse in the care of handicapped children.

The school meals service is particularly involved where special diets are needed as an essential part of the treatment of some conditions, such as coeliac disease.

```
                  The education department
        1   A local authority department
        2   Responsible for educational provisions
        3   Also provides:
               School psychological service
               Education social work service
               Child care assistants
               School meals service
```

Voluntary bodies

Many voluntary agencies offer help to children and their families by making provisions of a kind not covered by the statutory services, or which supplement them. The range of services provided is enormous, and may include:

1 Information and advice about a particular disorder or social problem, and facilities for help; this is particularly useful to the children themselves as they get older, as well as to the parents, and also helps to increase public understanding.
2 Opportunities for parents to meet together to exchange information and discuss common problems.
3 Social activities for young children, particularly the handicapped.
4 Special welfare workers who help families with specific problems.
5 Fund-raising to finance research, give financial assistance where necessary, provide holidays and special residential homes.
6 Acting as pressure groups to focus public attention on areas of concern, improve services and change existing laws.

The part played by voluntary agencies is extremely valuable and all professional workers in the children's services should be aware of what help can be obtained through them.

Co-ordinated care

The wide range of services within the Health Service itself, together with those provided by other statutory departments and voluntary agencies, underline the need for co-ordination of care in order to avoid overlap or omission and to prevent confusion brought about by conflicting advice. The need for integrated care becomes very apparent in the management of some childhood disorders. Handicap is probably an outstanding example, and will be discussed in Chapter 10; malignant disease is mentioned in Chapter 3. Three other conditions which also illustrate the need for co-ordinated care are diabetes, asthma, and epilepsy.

Diabetes

This condition occurs when the pancreas fails to produce sufficient insulin for the metabolism of sugar. Diabetes may occur at any age. The principal symptoms are:

1 Vague general symptoms of tiredness, irritability and 'not feeling well'.
2 Failure to thrive—there may often be a marked weight loss.

3 Abdominal pain.
4 Polyuria; diabetes should be considered as a possible reason for secondary enuresis in a child who has previously achieved bladder control.
5 Unusual thirst.

Glucose is present in the urine, and a random blood-sugar estimation may show an abnormally high glucose concentration.

> *Treatment*: This involves the administration of insulin usually by injection, although the type used, its dosage and frequency varies from child to child. A special diet is necessary, in which the carbohydrate content is controlled. Enough food must be taken to supply bodily requirements, including fibre intake, and the carbohydrate ration is usually spread evenly throughout the day; mid-morning and mid-afternoon snacks are often included in the dietary programme.

When the prescribed treatment is followed, general progress is satisfactory. Diabetic coma is rare, but hypoglycaemic attacks due to a sudden fall in blood-sugar are more common and tend to occur before meals, when a snack is forgotten, or during exercise. The child may become irritable, pale, sweaty and sleepy, but responds to sugar; all diabetic children should carry sugar lumps or sweets with them.

Asthma

Asthma is a condition in which episodes of dyspnoea and wheezing occur as a result of the lower airways becoming obstructed. In young children under the age of three, a virus respiratory infection usually precedes the asthmatic attack; in older children emotional factors, some forms of exercise, cold air, smoky atmosphere or allergy (particularly to house dust or domestic animals) may also precipitate an attack. It is estimated that about 5 % of all children suffer from asthma.

> *Treatment*: This varies according to the age of the child, the frequency and severity of attacks, and the extent to which normal home and school life are being interrupted. In mild infrequent attacks, bronchodilator drugs such as salbutamol can be given orally for the duration of the attack. When they are more frequent or severe, however, prophylactic therapy often is considered. This takes the form of the inhalation of intal (sodium cromoglycate) through a spinhaler, which must be used four times a day. A rotahaler enables bronchodilators or steroid preparations to be taken in a similar way. Special instructions to the child in the use of inhalers are needed, and to obtain a good response they must be used during school hours as well as at home.

Steroids can also be given in a pressurised aerosol, the use of which again needs practice and patience on the part of the parent and child. Children under the age of three or four find difficulty in mastering inhalation techniques and oral steroids may be prescribed for them, and for children not responding to other forms of prophylaxis. Steroid dosage needs careful balance in order to avoid side-effects, particularly growth restriction.

Epilepsy

This is a condition characterised by 'fits' or 'seizures' which result from alteration in the electrical activity of the brain. There are many forms of epilepsy, some of which arise from known causes, others in which the origin is obscure. The fits vary in severity from the classical picture of loss of consciousness, accompanied by stiffening and jerky movements of the limbs, to attacks of 'petit mal' where there is only a momentary loss of awareness. The diagnosis of epilepsy is made on the history and description of a fit, followed by physical and neurological examination, and investigations which include various forms of skull X-ray, electroencephalography (EEG) and biochemical tests. It is estimated that 8 in every 1000 school children have epilepsy, and probably many more will have had a fit at some time in their life.

Treatment: Once the type of epilepsy has been defined, its control depends upon the administration of anti-convulsant drugs and the avoidance of any factors known to trigger off an attack in an individual child. Drug therapy, both in type and dosage, is carefully chosen so as to maintain control of the fits and avoid or minimise any untoward side-effects such as behaviour disturbances, learning difficulties or undue drowsiness.

The management of diabetes, asthma and epilepsy Though obviously very different in their medical context, these three conditions have some aspects in common where their management is concerned.

The hospital usually undertakes the initial diagnosis, assessment, prescription of appropriate treatment, discussion with parents and follow-up procedures, but for the most part these children are living at home and attending school within the community, although from time to time brief periods of in-patient care may be needed. The primary care team, pre-school and school health services need information about recommendations made by the hospital staff and, similarly, the hospital staff need to be aware of the response to suggested therapy, particularly if this is not proving as effective as anticipated.

The responsibility for seeing that the treatment is followed lies mainly with the parents, to a lesser extent with the school, and to an increasing extent with the child as he grows older. Even after preliminary discussion at the hospital, repeated advice and reassurance are often necessary in the practical side of treatment, such as the giving of injections, testing of urine, use of inhalers, minor adjustments of therapy and diet, and dealing with emergency situations. Help in such aspects of care should be available from within the community services.

Total care also involves the emotional and social aspects of a child's life. Once a disorder has been diagnosed, the family may experience a period during which adjustments must be made if life is to continue as normally as possible. Different feelings are experienced of shock, resentment, guilt, anxiety and isolation. Parents and children need people within the community to whom they can turn for support and reassurance on a repeated and long-term basis; this may be met by the general practitioner, family or specialist health visitor, social worker, home nurse, school nurse or welfare worker from a specialised association.

School life must continue on as normal a basis as possible; knowledge of the likely effects of such disorders on educational progress is as much a part of total care as medical treatment. The school health service can help and support teachers and educational psychologists in educating them about the nature of the disorder, principles of treatment, possible bearing on school and behavioural progress, and the necessity to provide a normal school environment. Discussion of the progress of individual children between paediatrician, school health service staff, general practitioner and teacher is important.

A specialist health visitor, home nurse, or a paediatric nurse working in both the hospital and community can have an important role in the co-ordination of services and improvement of patterns of care for children with diabetes, severe asthma or epilepsy. She can maintain up-to-date knowledge on treatment and the services available, and act as a 'resource person' for other community staff in the primary care team, the school health service and education services, being herself helped and supported by the hospital staff with whom she has frequent contact about individual children. Her intimate knowledge of the child and his family would enable them to regard her as their source of advice, guidance and reassurance, thus improving the quality of their life and reducing the number of hospital visits and demands on general practitioner time.

In general, co-ordination of care is encouraged by:

1 Planning of health services in conjunction, where appropriate, with other agencies such as the education and social services departments. The Joint Consultative Committee of the health and local authorities and its special planning groups operate on these principles and can consider ways of improving the delivery of health care.

2   Workers being aware of and understanding each other's roles and functions and the type of service offered by different agencies. This applies on a general basis, and particularly to the contribution to total care in individual situations.

3   Good communication between individual professional workers so that, as far as possible, relevant information is shared. Transfer of information accurately, quickly and within the limits of confidentiality is not always simple. Telephone conversations, letters and case conferences have their place, and the development of a simple health record book (held by the parents) in which entries about the child's progress are made by the different professional workers involved in the child's care could be useful.

Co-ordinated care

1   Is essential to secure the best treatment for children and help for parents
2   Needs careful planning at local and national levels
3   Involves all workers in an understanding of each other's role
4   Demands good communication between professionals

The future

The Court report 'Fit for the Future' published in 1976 critically examined the child health services and made recommendations for future developments. The report emphasises the need for a service which is child- and family-centred and envisages a continuum of care in which surveillance, preventive health and care of the sick child are undertaken by the primary care worker, rather than being, as now, a responsibility split amongst pre-school clinics, the school health service, general practitioner and community nursing staff, who may also have duties with other groups of the population. Such an integrated service would encourage the development of paediatric professional skills in the community and enable parents to identify a single service which would give all forms of primary care and thus avoid the confusion which sometimes, at present, exists in distinguishing the functions of the separate services and using them appropriately. The specific recommendation that some general practitioners (general practitioner paediatricians) and health visitors (child health visitors) should concentrate exclusively on children and their families in health and sickness has not been accepted by the professional bodies concerned, although many general practitioners are including preventive child health in their services, with some specialisation in this field within group practices.

The Court report, however, has succeeded in stimulating attempts at greater integration of hospital and community services, and better communication between them. There is increasing interchange of hospital and community medical staff, sometimes in joint appointments and in the appointment of hospital liaison health visitors and specialist health visitors. The importance of services being easily available to all families was also stressed in the report and has resulted in critical appraisal of existing services, identification of barriers between family and service, and ways of improving facilities so that they are acceptable to the would-be users, particularly those families for whom they would appear to be most valuable.

10
Children with Handicap

The great majority of children grow and develop normally to lead a fully independent adult life, but others are born with, or later develop, disabling conditions which may cause handicap. Handicap can take many forms:

1 *Physical handicap* arising from, for example, loss or absence of a limb, abnormality of movement as in cerebral palsy, paralysis as in some forms of spina bifida, or from severe chronic disease such as asthma.
2 *Sensory handicap* such as blindness or deafness.
3 *Mental handicap* may present as an entity by itself, or may form part of a specific syndrome such as Down's syndrome (Mongolism) or be a feature of some (but not all) cases of spina bifida and cerebral palsy.
4 *Emotional handicap* is not always as immediately obvious as physical or mental handicap. It occurs when the child's emotional development is delayed or distorted, with the result that he reacts and behaves in abnormal ways.
5 *Social handicap* shows in the inability to achieve the degree of independence and social relationships expected of a particular age.

Although one aspect of handicap may predominate in an individual child, there is often a combination of two or more forms. A child with a physical handicap caused by spina bifida or cerebral palsy may also have sensory defects and mental retardation. Emotional and social handicaps are frequently linked and may also add another dimension to a physical or mental handicap.

Handicap takes many forms

1 It can affect the physical, mental, sensory, emotional and social aspects of development
2 One handicap may predominate, but often other forms are also present

---

Prevention of handicap

Prevention involves a recognition of the many different causative factors underlying the various forms of handicap, a knowledge of the times at ·

which the child is most vulnerable to their influence, and the means by which their potentially harmful effects can be overcome or minimised. The promotion of good health in children is the basic concern of the preventive child health services, and the ways in which factors associated with handicap can be detected and counteracted have already been discussed in previous chapters. They include:

1 Genetic counselling where there is a risk of disabling conditions caused by the inheritance of harmful genes or chromosome abnormalities.
2 Ensuring good maternal health at the time of conception.
3 Early and regular attendance for ante-natal supervision, together with high standards of obstetric care which facilitate:

   (a) Screening procedures such as blood tests, amniocentesis and ultrasound.
   (b) Detection of complications of pregnancy.

4 Health education programmes:

   (a) During pregnancy, to encourage mothers to adopt measures which minimise the risk of handicap—a balanced diet, no smoking, limited alcohol consumption, and the use of pre-scribed drugs only.
   (b) Helping parents to be aware of ways in which health and development of the child can be encouraged.

5 Care of the new-born, especially those of low birth weight, followed by programmes of health and developmental surveillance.
6 Immunisation programmes, particularly against poliomyelitis and rubella.
7 The early recognition and treatment of illness such as meningitis.
8 A general recognition of the needs of the child for a healthy and safe environment.

Prevention of handicap

1   Genetic counselling
2   Good maternal health
3   High standards of ante-natal and neo-natal care
4   Health education for parents
5   Surveillance programmes
6   Immunisation procedures
7   Early recognition of illness
8   A good environment

Some forms of handicap still persist either because, as yet, the cause remains obscure, or because preventive measures have not been fully effective. The aim here is to ensure, as far as possible, a good quality of life for child and family. A handicapped child has all the needs of a normal child for love, affection, security, material care, stimulus and education but, in addition, often requires specialised help from many different sources—health and local authority services, voluntary associations and individual members of the community. In order to be able to give maximum help to the handicapped child and his family, it is necessary:

1 To identify them—who they are and where they are.
2 To assess the extent of the handicap.
3 To remedy what can be remedied, and institute measures to minimise the degree of residual handicap.
4 To re-assess at intervals, recognising that needs change.
5 To give, at all times, support and assistance to child and family.

The identification of handicapped children

It is important that a child with an obvious handicap, or with a suspected one, is recognised at the earliest possible stage in order to begin appropriate treatment, therapy, advice and counselling at the most advantageous time.

Notification of congenital abnormalities

The presence of a congenital defect obvious at the time of birth is indicated on the birth notification form, so that community health staff (doctor, midwife and health visitor) are aware of the condition and can be satisfied that any further investigation or treatment is in hand. Not all congenital defects lead to permanent handicap. Some are very minor defects, causing no disability; some may be corrected by medical treatment or surgical procedures. Others, however, such as Down's syndrome, severe forms of spina bifida and microcephaly, will signify a degree of permanent handicap.

Programmes of surveillance

Surveillance of growth, physical health, development and educational progress will help to identify those children with:

1 Congenital defects not clinically apparent at birth
2 Disorders becoming recognisable as development proceeds

3 Difficulties in learning
4 Social and emotional problems

It is important to remember that amidst all the professional staff involved in programmes of surveillance, the parents may be the first people to recognise that all is not well.

Information about intercurrent events

Unforeseen incidents in the child's life, such as unexpected illness or injury, sudden changes in the home and social environment likely to result in handicap, may come to the notice of any one of the professional workers in contact with the child and family—consultant, general practitioner, health visitor, community child health doctor, social worker or teacher. It is important that the significance of these events is recognised, and relevant information passed on to those who would be specially involved in future assessment and management.

A register of handicapped children is compiled by many Health Authorities. It contains information about children who are likely to have a substantial degree of permanent handicap for which special services will be needed, and is kept updated and under regular review by a senior community medical officer. The register is used:

1 For statistical and planning purposes.
2 As a means of follow-up of individual children to ensure the availability and co-ordination of necessary services.

The Health Authority has a statutory duty to inform the Local Education Authority of any child under the age of five who is considered to be so severely handicapped that special educational provisions will be needed. Before doing this, the matter must first of all be discussed with the parents at a stage when the prognosis for the child seems reasonably clear.

Identification of handicap

1 Notification of congenital abnormality
2 Programmes of surveillance
3 Observations of parents
4 Information about specific episodes of illness or injury

Initial assessment procedures

By whatever means identification is made of handicap or suspected handicap, a system should operate whereby further investigation can be carried out. This will vary in detail according to the type of handicap but, in all cases, its purpose is similar.

1 The full extent of the obvious or suspected handicap can be ascertained and, where possible, its cause identified. This enables the parents to be given some explanation and, where appropriate, advised to seek genetic counselling to help them in the planning of future pregnancies.

2 Other handicaps can be identified. The presenting handicap is sometimes not the only one; others not so easily recognisable occur in association and handicap in one field of development often secondarily affects development in other aspects.

3 It enables the child's handicap to be seen in the context of the whole child, his family and social background. The degree of handicap which a disability causes is not totally determined by the medical aspects of the condition, but is influenced by the child's intelligence and personality, and by his environment at home and in school.

4 A programme of management can be mapped out for each child, which will include any treatment considered to be necessary, arrangements for family support and suggestions about the child's educational needs.

5 A base-line can be established for future evaluation of progress. Assessment is not a once and for all procedure, but rather a series of observations and tests carried out at intervals.

Depending on the type of disability and handicap, the procedures which assessment involves vary considerably. General practitioners or community child health doctors carry out a preliminary assessment and may then decide to refer the child for more detailed investigation:

1 For some children, examination in a specialised unit is indicated— for example, investigation in a cardio-thoracic unit or at a haemophilia reference centre.

2 In school children with learning or behavioural difficulties, initial assessment often involves teachers, the educational psychologist, school doctor and nurse, who may later decide that a full multi-professional assessment or referral to the child psychiatric service is needed.

3 In young pre-school children, particularly those with severe disability or multiple handicap, assessment is ideally carried out by a multi-disciplinary team, each member of which can contribute individual expertise to help build up a complete picture.

The multi-disciplinary handicap team

This team forms a pool from which expertise can be drawn as seems most appropriate for the type of disability and the age of the child. It includes:

The consultant paediatrician, with special experience in the field of handicap and who may be a paediatric neurologist.

The community medical officer, also with a special knowledge of handicap in children (particularly from the educational aspect) who is aware of the range and availability of community provisions and has links with the services providing them.

The physiotherapist, who assesses the physical condition of the child from the aspect of posture, movements and balance, and can help the child towards achieving active independence by means of suitable exercises.

The occupational therapist, who is concerned with the child's ability to play constructively and to perform activities of daily living appropriate to his age (for example in feeding, dressing, washing) and who encourages the child to use his hands and arms, and gives advice regarding suitable toys and home equipment.

The speech therapist, who assesses speech and language development and the child's ability to communicate. Observation during a meal will give information about swallowing and chewing as a pre-requisite of speech development.

The audiometrician, who assesses hearing and the ability to distinguish different sounds.

The orthoptist, responsible for testing vision and detecting any defects such as squint.

The psychologist, who is concerned with measuring intelligence, assessing personality and, by skilled counselling of child and family, tries to resolve stresses before they develop into serious problems.

Assessment teachers, who understand the need for learning through play and, together with the physiotherapist and occupational therapist, develop various activities for the child.

Nursing staff, who look after the general needs of the child and his parents. In the course of helping to smooth their passage through the multiplicity of procedures, they make their own observations on the child's abilities and behaviour, and on the parents' attitudes and reactions.

The medical social worker and *liaison* or *specialist health visitor*, who are particularly concerned with the home and social environment of the child. They are able to contribute a great deal of information about the parents—their intelligence, feelings, attitudes and expectations for their handicapped child. They also know something of the material conditions of the home and any difficulties the family may be experiencing regarding finance, housing or practical help, and can give an impression of the culture and attitudes of the community in which the family live. Their assessment of the family is very important in enabling a plan of therapy to be instituted which, because it takes into account particular difficulties, is realistic and within the capacity of the parents to accept.

The parents, whose knowledge and observations of their own child are invaluable and who should be regarded as essential participants in assessment.

The assessment team may also include (as the occasion demands for individual children) the family doctor, school doctor, family health visitor and social worker, who not only provide additonal details from their own knowledge of the child but are able to gain first-hand information of the degree of handicap and the proposals made for therapy. The consultants in dentistry, orthopaedics, ophthalmology and child psychiatry may be involved in the full assessment of some particular types of handicap.

The multi-disciplinary handicap team

1 Consultant paediatrician
2 Community medical officer
3 Therapists—physio, occupational and speech
4 Audiometrician
5 Orthoptist
6 Psychologist
7 Assessment teachers
8 Nursing staff
9 Medical social workers and specialist health visitors
10 Parents

The core of the multi-disciplinary team is usually based in the assessment unit and the initial assessment may take several days to complete. Arrangements are made for daily transport of child and parents, or alternatively for over-night stay. A preliminary home visit by the team medical social worker or health visitor is very helpful in explaining to the parents the programme of the assessment and the various procedures involved. Although some parts of the assessment are, of necessity, carried out in a special unit, members of the team are aware that a great deal can be learned from watching the child in everyday situations such as the home, school, day nursery or playgroup, and are prepared to extend their activities out into the community.

Therapy and management

At the end of the assessment procedures each member of the team presents his findings and makes recommendations to be incorporated into a future plan of management. This differs widely from child to child according to the type and degree of handicap, but is essentially a 'prescription for action' which indicates ways in which provisions should be made for treatment and therapy in different forms and sequences. As far as practicable, the aim is for these programmes to be maintained in the community. Consequently, advice about the child's capabilities and needs should be given to the people who will be most concerned with his future care—his family, general practitioner, health visitor, social worker, school doctor and nurse, and teachers. The 'prescription for action' includes, as necessary:

1 *Medical or surgical treatment*, for instance the control of epileptic fits, orthopaedic operations, procedures to relieve urinary incontinence and facilities for the treatment of emergency situations.

2 *Dental treatment.* Many children, particularly those with cerebral palsy or mental retardation, need special dental care.

3 *Help with emotional difficulties*, which often become more pronounced as the child grows older and realises the limitations imposed by his handicap.

4 *Programmes of therapy* to develop independence in the fields of locomotion and manipulation. These may require regular attendance at a special unit but should, where possible, be suitable for continuation at home. Parents are encouraged to participate in therapy supported by home visits from the assessment team members, or by enlisting the help of therapists working in the community. Similarly, the speech therapist indicates to the parents ways in which they can encourage language development.

5 *The provision of aids* such as glasses, hearing aids, splints, calipers and frames.

6 *Discussion*, frank and unhurried, with the parents to explain the nature of the handicap, the proposed plan of action, to answer their questions, to explore their needs and put them in touch with other services which could give additional help.

7 *Sending a report* of the findings and recommendations to other professionals involved in the care of the child and his family.

> *A 'prescription for action'*
>
> 1 Medical or surgical treatment where necessary
> 2 Dental treatment
> 3 Help with emotional difficulties
> 4 Encouragement of independence
> 5 Provision of aids
> 6 Discussion with parents
> 7 Reports to others involved with care of the child

Ongoing assessment

Re-assessment at intervals is necessary in order to judge the results of a suggested programme, after allowing a reasonable time for it to become effective and for interim reports of progress from health visitors, doctors or teachers to be considered. As the child is enabled to develop his potential through the intervention programme, so his needs will change and different patterns of therapy and services will then be required so as to maintain maximum improvement. Re-assessment is concerned not only with identifying the changing needs of the child, but also with a new look at his environment. Within the family, material circumstances fluctuate and, more importantly, parents' attitudes alter either in response to change in the child or through the counselling and support they themselves have received. Special assessment is needed to decide the most appropriate form of education (page 195). During school life itself, response to one form of education may be such that some variation is needed and hence a whole range of facilities enables a flexible programme to be maintained.

Re-assessment is particularly important at the time of adolescence when new aspects of handicap emerge, such as the question of transfer to the adult hospital system, the parents' attitudes (which sometimes change with the prospect of caring for an adult rather than a child) and the emotional problems of the child himself, for which special counselling may be needed.

> *Help for the child with a handicap*
>
> 1 Identification
> 2 Initial assessment procedures
> 3 Therapy and management
> 4 Ongoing assessment
> 5 Practical support of child and family

Support for child, parents and family

Parents are the mainstay of care for the majority of handicapped children and, in their turn, often require a great deal of help, both in the form of counselling and practical assistance, to enable them to meet their child's needs.

1 Counselling

Getting to know about handicap

Counselling is an ongoing process starting when the parents first suspect or become aware of handicap and recognising that changing situations bring different needs. One of the most difficult and distressing situations for both parents and professional staff arises when the news is first broken to the parents. Depending on the nature of the disability producing the handicap, the time at which the subject is raised varies. Congenital defects likely to cause considerable handicap are usually very obvious at birth and indicate early discussion, particularly when urgent decisions may have to be made about management. This is a time of great emotional upheaval for both parents and they should be told by a senior doctor with a sensitive appreciation of their feelings, who can explain the siutation simply and honestly. The ward nursing staff, through their own caring attitude and sharing of grief, are able to help the mother through the first difficult days when, in spite of her own distress, she must begin her relationship with her child. The medical social worker is another person to whom parents may turn for comfort and advice; in some maternity units special health visitors or social workers are appointed to be involved in the initial counselling and provide continuity after the mother returns home.

Handicaps which arise later should be discussed with the parents by the general practitioner and paediatric consultant and sometimes this is best done in several stages. A positive approach should be adopted, stressing what is possible in the way of achievement and sources of help, but keeping within the bounds of reality. Many parents find it impossible to realise straightaway the full implications of the information they have been given and for varying periods of time afterwards will repeatedly seek explanation from many different people. It is important for professional staff in the community to be aware of the diagnosis and of what the parents have been told so that their counselling and advice will reinforce what has already been given. At an appropriate stage simple explanatory books and leaflets are often helpful for the parents to read.

Continuing counselling

Many parents of a handicapped child at first feel that their experience is unique and their consequent embarrassment keeps them apart from other people. Isolation adds to the risk of depression. Parents need someone in whom they feel they can confide their true feelings of anger, grief and guilt—a person with time, patience, understanding and an awareness of their problems and possible sources of additional help. This person may vary at different times—it could be the health visitor, general practitioner, social worker, clinic doctor or advisory teacher. The family or specialist health visitor will give assistance in the early days about feeding and general care, advice about the general needs of all children, and the special needs of this particular child. Therapy today lays stress on enlisting the help of parents in the encouragement of the child's development and this, in turn, helps them to develop confidence. Some gain a great deal of support by joining a group of parents of children with similar handicaps and thus being able share their feelings, difficulties and triumphs with each other.

Special counselling

Circumstances may arise in connection with specific handicapping conditions or relationships within the family which indicate the need for special help:

1 Dilemmas of choice   Some congenital defects, by reason either of their nature or severity, present dilemmas to both parents and medical and nursing staff. Spina bifida is a case in point, where sensitive and careful counselling is needed not only to comfort parents in their initial distress, but also to help them understand the reasons for and against early intervention and to support them in whatever decision they make on their child's behalf. There has been a great deal of recent debate on the subject of deliberately keeping alive children for whom their parents feel there is very little future, even though with medical and surgical intervention life could be prolonged indefinitely. This is a very complex issue, involving not only medical ethics but legal, religious and moral principles, and all these aspects may need to be discussed at some time during the counselling process.

2 Genetic counselling   It is possible to obtain expert information about the likelihood of specific harmful genes and chromosome abnormalities being passed on. The general practitioner, clinic doctor or hospital consultant is often able to explain to parents what the chances are, but sometimes further referral to a special centre for genetic counselling is advisable. Genetic counselling should be specially considered:

(a)   When a child in the family develops an illness or handicapping condition thought to be due totally or partially to inherited factors, such as cystic fibrosis, Down's syndrome and spina bifida.

(b)   When there is a history of inherited illness or abnormality in the family and parents may wish to know whether there is a chance of the disease developing in themselves or in any children they may have.

(c)   When an abnormal condition can be detected in early pregnancy. Discussion can be arranged about the availability of special antenatal tests and possible termination of pregnancy.

(d)   Where marital partners are closely related.

A genetic counsellor needs a precise diagnosis of the condition about which he is being consulted, together with the medical and family history of the child and parents. An examination of the chromosome make-up of the child and parents may be indicated and is usually carried out on a blood sample. When all the information has been assembled, the counsellor is able to explain how the condition has arisen and can estimate the chances of it appearing in a subsequent child, or in children of a following generation. Once the counsellor feels that his clients understand the information he has given, any decisions about future pregnancies are usually left with them, although they should be made aware of family planning facilities.

3   Family crises   Many parents gradually adjust to the changes which a handicap in a child brings, particularly if adequate counselling and practical help has been available. Sometimes, however, a great deal of stress arises in family life and may threaten the stability of the marriage. Perceptive counselling uncovers difficulties in relationships and adjustment or problems of mental health in one or both parents which may need referral for more specialised advice and therapy.

4   Siblings   Counselling aimed at helping the family as a whole recognises that brothers and sisters of a handicapped child may need special help in resolving some of their own personal difficulties. One child may feel resentful that his parents' attention and time is focused on his handicapped sibling, another a heavy responsibility that parents' expectations of a successful normal child are now centred on him. Other children, as they grow older, feel embarrassment about the appearance or behaviour of their handicapped sibling, are unwilling to bring their friends home and, in consequence, their social life becomes restricted. A school or family counsellor will recognise their difficulties, encourage them to share their feelings, and help parents to appreciate the need for balance in meeting the needs of their other children as well as those of the handicapped child.

5 Home or residential care The great majority of parents feel deeply that they wish to care for their handicapped child at home for as long as possible, but circumstances may arise which make home care extremely difficult, if not impossible—for instance, when a parent is ill, handicapped or alone, or when accompanying behaviour problems (particularly in the older handicapped child) are completely disrupting family life. Parents may need a great deal of wise counselling to enable them to accept that alternative care is necessary. Increasing importance is being placed on the need for short-term residential provisions which relieve an urgent situation and enable the decision regarding permanent care to be postponed.

6 Problems in an adolescent handicapped child Handicapped children approaching adolescence and adulthood have special counselling needs in their own right. They often need help in coming to terms with the limitations which their handicap imposes on their social life, prospects of a career and adult independence. Special anxieties arise about sexual matters—their ability to enjoy a full sexual relationship, and doubts about the possibility and practicality of marriage and parenthood. Many different people may be able to help them, such as parents, school teaching and pastoral staff, school health service staff and social workers. Some family planning clinics offer counselling from staff with special experience in the sexual difficulties associated with some forms of handicap, but this is a field in which a great deal more provision could be made. Parents may express concern about a mentally handicapped child who is unable to understand the physical and emotional changes of adolescence and, in the case of a girl, may become exposed to the risk of an unwanted pregnancy. Discussion with the general practitioner or a family planning doctor will enable suggestions to be made on practical management and appropriate contraceptive measures to be arranged.

Counselling for parents

1 Telling about handicap in the child
2 Insight into feelings
3 Special counselling:
    Dilemmas of choice
    Genetic counselling
    Family crises
    Siblings
    Home or residential care
    Adolescent problems

2 Practical support for the family

A wide range of practical provisions are needed to make life easier and more rewarding for child and family alike. Such help may make all the difference to the ability of the family to cope, to be able to keep the child at home, and in the prevention or relief of stress. Not only is the provision of services necessary, but information should be widely publicised about their existence, their purpose and how they may be obtained. The health visitor or the specialist health visitor, working in conjunction with the assessment team, has been suggested as the 'named person' to whom parents of young children can turn, not only for counselling but also as the community worker who is able to discuss their practical needs and put them in touch with available services. During school life the 'named person' would probably be the head teacher or a designated member of staff whom the parents could easily contact for advice. It is helpful to issue booklets giving comprehensive information about local, as well as general, services for children with special needs, so that parents and young handicapped people themselves have, at all times, an easily accessible source of reference.

Finance

Care of a handicapped child often involves the parents in additional expense; extra heating may be necessary, special clothing and bedding needed, additional washing is incurred and, in some instances, mothers who would otherwise be augmenting the family income must either stay at home to look after the child or pay for the services of a child-minder. A number of benefits are available:

The attendance allowance is a non-contributory tax-free weekly benefit payable to, or on behalf of, people (including children over the age of two) who are so severely mentally or physically disabled that a great deal of additional help is needed to attend to their physical needs, or to prevent them harming themselves or other people. This allowance is designed to give the parents some relief from the continual care of their child and is payable at higher or lower rates, depending on whether care is needed day and night or for only part of the 24 hours. Explanatory leaflets and claim forms are available from social security offices.

The mobility allowance enables parents of children over the age of five years, who are unable (or almost unable) to walk because of their physical handicap, to receive a tax-free weekly benefit. It helps parents in the payment of taxi fares for transport of the child to social activities, on day outings or holidays, and so enables the child's horizons to be expanded and his experience of the outside world increased.

Free milk is available for handicapped children aged five to sixteen years who are not attending school.

Free transport to and from school is arranged by most education authorities.

The Family Fund is set up by the Government, and administered by the Joseph Rowntree Memorial Trust. It provides, for the families of severely handicapped children, help of a type that is not normally covered by the statutory services. The assistance given is usually in kind rather than in money (for instance, the provision of a washing machine, clothing, bedding, television for the house-bound, and holidays) although a sum of money may be allotted for a specific purpose such as car purchase or hire, or driving lessons for parents. The social services department will give information on how the fund can be contacted.

Voluntary organisations and charitable trusts may be able to give help in money or kind.

Financial help

1 Constant attendance allowance
2 Mobility allowance
3 Free milk
4 Free transport to school
5 The Family Fund
6 Assistance from voluntary organisations

Housing

Good housing conditions for the handicapped child are extremely important. While the child is small and can easily be carried about housing requirements are similar to those of any parents with a young family, but as he gets older and bigger the situation changes. Where a wheelchair is needed, space may be limited and access difficult. Steep, winding stairs present a formidable obstacle to the parent struggling with a heavy adolescent. Toilet facilities may be inconvenient and inadequate. The housing and social services departments of the local authority work closely together to find solutions to these difficulties:

1 Many housing departments give priority on medical grounds for rehousing in more suitable accommodation, such as bungalows and ground-floor flats.

2 Improvement grants can make it possible for some existing houses to be made more suitable for a handicapped child—for instance, in the provision of a bathroom and indoor toilet.
3 Minor adaptations to the house, such as widening of doorways, building of ramps to make wheelchair access easier, the provision of handrails, special toilets and showers, are the responsibility of the social services department.

Help in housing

1 Priority for rehousing
2 Improvement grants
3 Home adaptations

Aids for daily living

There are several aids which help the child towards achieving some degree of independence in dressing, toileting and feeding. The social services department and the British Red Cross Society supply a wide range of special equipment such as crockery, cutlery, toilet and dressing aids. The District Health Authority provides nursing equipment for use in the home, varying from special feeding cups to hoists. The authority also arranges for the distribution and disposal of incontinence pads for use in bed, and rolls for use with incontinence pants.

Mobility

When it is thought that a physical handicap is likely to be permanent, various mobility aids are available through the DHSS on the recommendation of a medical practitioner. These include wheelchairs, pushchairs and tricycles, all of which should be carefully selected so as best to meet individual requirements.

Leisure activities

In the same way that normal children need leisure-time pursuits, so too do handicapped children, to an equal if not greater extent. Not only do such activities give a great deal of enjoyment, but they are also invaluable in stimulating development and should be regarded as an essential part of life. A wide range of activities is available through the education and social services departments and voluntary organisations, including facilities for swimming, riding, social clubs, day-outings and longer holidays. Organised play during school holidays gives the opportunity for handicapped children to mix with other children.

Parents also need to have some leisure time to pursue their own interests; many voluntary organisations provide social activities for them and make arrangements for 'baby' sitters. The social services department provides facilities for short-term residential care for the handicapped child to enable parents and other children in the family to have a holiday together.

Facilities for day care

Occasions arise when day care is needed to relieve the situation when:

1 The mother is obliged to go out to work.
2 The continued strain of caring for a severely handicapped child is becoming too great.
3 The mother is mentally or physically ill, or is otherwise unable to give her child adequate care and stimulation at home.

Provisions include:

Day nurseries, which are the responsibility of the social services department and will be discussed in detail in the next chapter. Special nurseries for handicapped children may be provided but many ordinary day nurseries accept a small number of handicapped children. The day nursery relieves the mother of care for part or whole of the day and also encourages social development and learning through play, linking closely with the assessment unit and the education department.

Child-minders, who offer an alternative form of day care, whereby the mother arranges to leave her child in the minder's home, and pays for this service. Child-minders must be registered with the social services department, and those undertaking care of a handicapped child should have an understanding of the child's needs, particularly as she may be taking over the parents' role in providing home therapy.

Home helps, who may be provided by the social services department in special circumstances to enable the mother to give sufficient time and care to her child.

Day care facilities

1 Day nursery
2 Child-minder
3 Home help

Full-time care

A range of accommodation is available for 24-hour care over varying periods of time; this is provided by the health authority or the social services department, depending on the amount of nursing care the child needs. Short-stay facilities cater for a variety of circumstances:

1 Some offer overnight stay for one or two nights a week, giving the parents an opportunity to rest if their handicapped child has serious sleep problems.
2 Five-day units enable children to be resident during the weekdays, attending school from the unit and returning home for the weekends.
3 Short-stay home or hospital beds enable parents to have a holiday, or simply to renew their capacity to care for the child.

On a long-term basis, permanent care may be needed when the parents are no longer able to cope with their child, or when parental care is inadequate to the extent that the child's well-being is suffering. Facilities for long-stay care include:

1 Long-stay hospitals.
2 Hostel accommodation for adolescents.
3 Residential nurseries and community homes.
4 Fostering, in which the child is looked after in the foster parents' home by a couple approved by the social services department. Because of the needs of a handicapped child, such foster parents need exceptional qualities to enable them to carry out their task successfully and, in instances of temporary breakdown of parental care, to work alongside the social worker in helping to re-integrate the child into the family. Foster parents are being increasingly employed in a very flexible capacity to cover periods of time ranging from a few hours or several days to long-term care.

Full-time care

1 Short-stay:
    Overnight
    5-day units
    Short-stay home or hospital
2 Long-term:
    Hospital or hostel accommodation
    Residential nursery or community home
    Foster home

> *Practical support for the family*
> 1 Financial help
> 2 Housing
> 3 Aids for daily living
> 4 Mobility
> 5 Leisure activities
> 6 Facilities for day care
> 7 Full-time care

Education

The word 'education' is most commonly associated with formal school life, but taken in its true sense is to be regarded as a process of development of the powers of body and mind, which starts from the time of birth and in which formal schooling is part of the wider scene. For the very young child, the parents are the principal educators through their encouragement of the child by play, language, new experiences and introduction to a widening circle of people. Such opportunities are as important for the handicapped child as for the non-handicapped and parents should be involved from the earliest stage, understanding the role that they can play and being helped to achieve what is expected of them.

The Local Education Authority:
1 May appoint advisory teachers who, if the parents so wish, visit the home to advise on programmes of learning and help them develop the child's own skills.
2 Offers places in nursery schools or classes attached to ordinary and special schools.
3 May provide family centres which house toy libraries, display books and play material, and offer opportunities for parents to meet with professional staff.

Home visits may also be made by members of the district handicap team or the community therapists.

Play is encouraged through:
1 Toy libraries, where parents are advised on appropriate toys which they are able to borrow.
2 Attendance at a playgroup, which offers opportunities for children to mix with each other in creative play. Assessment units may include

a playgroup and many local groups accept a handicapped child. Other groups are specially organised for severely handicapped children and offer a gradual introduction to different forms of play.

Formal education

The Local Education Authority has a statutory duty to provide education for all children according to their age, aptitude and ability, and this includes those with 'learning difficulties giving rise to special educational needs'. In the educational context, the term 'learning difficulties' has now replaced the word 'handicap'.

Present-day policy on special educational needs has been largely influenced by the Warnock Report (1978) and some of its recommendations are embodied in the Education Act of 1981, indicating important areas of concern.

Where children with learning difficulties are concerned, the aim must be to promote education tailored, as far as possible, to the needs of the individual child (Fig. 10.1). This means that when a child with learning difficulties is identified his educational needs must be assessed. In the many instances where the difficulty is relatively small, the assessment will be an informal process undertaken by the teacher who recognises that adjustments will be possible within the existing school framework. When a child has a severe or complex disability, recognised either in the pre-school period or at school, a more formal assessment for special educational provision is considered, involving reports on the child's condition from teachers, educational psychologists, medical and nursing staff. The education department can then make a decision on the basis of the reports and, where necessary, inter-disciplinary discussion as to whether or not a statement of special educational needs is to be made with recommendations as to the type of education considered to be most suitable. The parents are informed of the assessment procedure and are sent a copy of the statement.

Wherever possible, children with learning difficulties of any degree should be educated within ordinary schools. This will mean considerable flexibility of educational methods (Fig. 10.2) and may involve adjustments to the physical layout of the school, such as wheelchair access, handrails and the staffing arrangements to include sufficient child care assistants. Extra support may be needed from physiotherapists, speech therapists and peripatetic teachers. The school doctor and nurse have an increasingly important role in reviewing the child's health, discussing progress with the teacher and in helping school staff to understand the nature of the child's disability in relation to educational needs.

When education in ordinary school is not considered to be in the best interests of the child, or would have a harmful effect on other children,

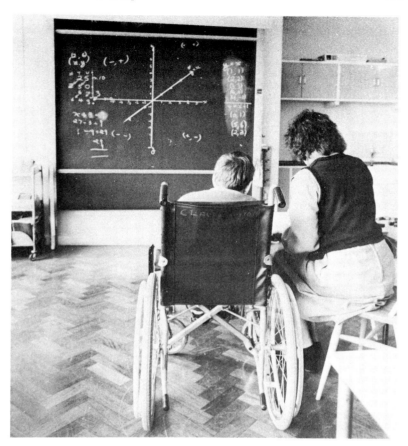

Fig. 10.1 Education tailored to need

he is recommended to a special school appropriate to his needs. There is a wide range of special schools catering for children with all forms of learning difficulty and often acting as resource centres for ordinary schools where a handicapped child is being educated.

Wherever possible it is preferable for children to attend school on a day basis, but sometimes unsuitable home conditions or travelling distance make residential school advisable. The education department also has a responsibility to arrange tuition for children who are in hospital for over two weeks (or for lesser periods if already attending special school) and for home tuition when attendance at school is absolutely impossible.

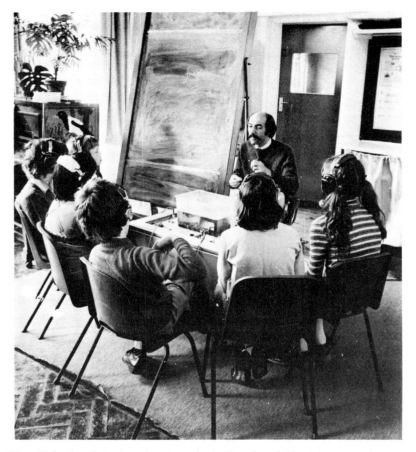

Fig. 10.2 Special educational methods for the child with severe hearing difficulty

The decision about placement in any school, ordinary or special, is not a rigid one and an annual review of the child's progress is essential. Provisions are sufficiently flexible to allow any child at any one time to receive the most suitable education for his needs, and so a change from ordinary school to special school and vice versa can be arranged.

A special assessment is recommended between the ages of 14 and 15 (i.e. about two years before the child is due to leave school) in order that his capabilities in relation to future work prospects can be estimated and careers' guidance given. This assessment procedure would include a careers officer.

Education

1 Starts from birth
2 Parents are educators
3 Pre-school provisions:
   Advisory teachers
   Nursery school
   Family centre
   Toy libraries
   Playgroups
4 Formal education:
   To meet individual needs
   In ordinary school where possible
   A flexible programme

Present and future

There appear to be two main issues in the consideration of handicap—prevention, and the planning of adequate services to meet the needs where handicap exists.

Prevention

A great deal has already been achieved in the reduction of some forms of handicap, and it is probable that even more will be possible in the future as improvements in perinatal care continue, and advances in genetic science increase the possibilities of pre-natal diagnosis of inherited conditions. In examining means of further prevention, two other aspects can be considered:

1 Although it is possible in some instances to point to one single factor which is responsible for a specific handicapping condition, very often many influences are operating and interweaving, some of which stem from social under-privilege.
2 In other instances, although the cause and prevention of handicap appear clear-cut, much depends on willingness to make use of services—for example, the uptake of facilities for rubella immunisation, and attendance for ante-natal care sufficiently early for alpha-feto protein estimation and amniocentesis to be of practical value.

Reduction of the incidence of handicap depends not only on the recognition of causes and designing appropriate preventive measures but in acknowledging the complexity of multiple factors, particularly the part played by social problems, and the need to influence people to take advantage of the services offered.

Planning of services

Over the years there has been a growth of many agencies with different forms of help to offer—the health service, education and social services departments, and voluntary societies. It is recognised that consultation and liaison at all levels are required, from case conferences on the needs of an individual child to joint planning exercises, such as take place in the Joint Consultative Committee and special planning groups. Planning at district level involves:

1 As far as is possible, a carefully calculated estimate, by local surveys, of the number of children already known to have a handicap and a forecast for the future in view of the anticipated degree of success of preventive measures.
2 Examination of existing services to ascertain how far they are meeting requirements.
3 Consideration of how the existing services could be adapted and expanded, what new services are needed to meet the basic needs of child and family, and their implication in terms of money, buildings, recruitment and training of staff.

In the same way that therapy changes the future needs of the individual child, so the provision and use of services change future requirements. Assessment and re-assessment of services are continually needed in order to ensure that children and their families are obtaining the help and support to enable them to live as full a life as possible.

Examples of handicap

Down's syndrome (Mongolism)

The inheritance of an extra chromosome number 21 gives rise to a number of developmental defects occurring together as Down's syndrome. These include:

1 A typical facial appearance in which there is a combination of slanting eyes, small nose, thick lips and a mouth apparently too small for the tongue which is constantly protruded.
2 Flabbiness of muscles which contributes to delay in walking.
3 Variable features of the hands and feet—a short incurved little finger and a wide cleft between first and second toes.

4 Mental retardation, which is always present but varies considerably in degree.
5 In the majority, a happy affectionate personality.
6 A proneness to respiratory infection and an increased association of other defects, particularly congenital heart disease and intestinal atresias.

The diagnosis is confirmed by chromosome analysis. It is important that the parents' chromosomes are also examined in order that they can be told of the chances of Down's syndrome occurring in a child of a subsequent pregnancy. Amniocentesis is offered to women over the age of 35 years who, because of their age, are at increased risk of producing a Mongol child, and to those where there is a previous history of a handicapped child; termination can be offered if a Down's syndrome fetus is identified. Remedial therapy helps a great deal in the encouragement of general development. Some Down's syndrome children achieve a good degree of independence in daily routines and are eventually able to undertake simple work, although the great majority will need some form of care throughout their lives.

Spina bifida (meningomyelocoele)

Spina bifida is a condition in which part of the spinal cord and the overlying vertebrae, muscles and skin fail to develop normally. It presents on the back as a plaque of immature nervous tissue protected only by a membrane. Depending on its position, spina bifida can cause:

1 Paralysis and loss of sensation in the lower limbs with later development of varying degrees of deformity.
2 Paralysis or incoordination of the bladder musculature causing incontinence and a risk of urinary infection and impaired renal function. There may also be faecal incontinence.
3 An increased risk of meningitis if the sac ruptures.

Spina bifida is often accompanied or followed by hydrocephalus, and visual defects, epilepsy, cerebral palsy and mental retardation are commonly associated disabilities. Spina bifida, in all but the very mild form known as 'spina bifida occulta', is obvious at the time of birth, and careful assessment of its severity is needed in order that a decision on the advisability of early intervention can be made, based on the likelihood of operation giving a reasonable quality of life for the future. Intervention procedures include closure of the back defect and the control of any associated or subsequent hydrocephalus, either by the insertion of a valve whereby excess cerebrospinal fluid is drained into the general circulation or, sometimes, by drug therapy. Later operations may be needed to correct limb deformities, scoliosis, and urinary and faecal incontinence.

The management of spina bifida involves the skill of many professionals working together as a team—the paediatrician, surgeon, orthopaedic consultant, psychologist and physiotherapist with, at times, the help of other specialists and community child health staff who mobilise and co-ordinate support services. The Association for Spina Bifida and Hydrocephalus offers help for spina bifida patients and their families; parent groups are encouraged, and holiday facilities for the children are available.

Genetic counselling is advised for parents who have already had a child with an abnormality of the central nervous system. Ante-natal screening by alpha-feto-protein estimation in the maternal blood and amniotic fluid (with subsequent termination of pregnancy where indicated) will reduce the incidence.

Mental retardation

This term is used to describe a condition in which almost every aspect of development is delayed, due to impairment of brain function. Some causes of mental retardation are known; it is a feature of specific disabilities such as Down's syndrome, or metabolic conditions such as untreated phenylketonuria or congenital hypothyroidism. Maternal infection with rubella in early pregnancy and post-natal infections in the child (such as meningitis and encephalitis) can cause mental retardation, and serious head injuries sometimes have a similar effect. In some instances there is a strong family history, but in many cases the underlying factor is obscure.

There are many degrees of mental retardation, varying from the relatively mild to those so severe that a fully independent life is impossible. An accurate estimate of the incidence is difficult but it is thought that at least 5 % of pre-school children will require special oversight. The main features of mental retardation are:

1   The baby is less alert, may sleep a lot, and takes little interest in his surroundings or toys.
2   Feeding problems arising from difficulty in sucking and learning to chew.
3   Delay in smiling, sitting, walking, developing skills of manipulation, speech and language. The latter tends to suffer more than other aspects of development, particularly in its use as a means of communication.
4   Difficulties in understanding and learning, which are particularly relevant to educational progress.

Early detection of mental retardation is important so as to enable a full assessment to be made and appropriate help for child and family arranged. The National Society for Mentally Handicapped Children

(MENCAP) looks after the interests of mentally handicapped children and their families; it supports local groups, tries to increase public understanding of the problem, and initiates research projects and innovations in care.

Cerebral palsy

This disorder results from damage to the developing brain, but there is still imprecise knowledge about its exact cause. In some instances an inherited factor is present, and events during the pre-natal period (such as maternal infection, pre-eclamptic toxaemia and placental malfunctioning) also contribute. It is known to be associated with immature gestation, anoxia before or during birth, and prolonged marked degrees of neo-natal jaundice. Meningitis, head injury and severe fits may also result in cerebral palsy. Its incidence is estimated to lie between 1 and 2 per 1000 live births.

The clinical picture varies a great deal in its form and severity. Signs of a severe degree of cerebral palsy are often detectable on the first-neo-natal examination; milder forms are identified by subsequent developmental screening.

1 Cerebral palsy may affect the arm and leg on one side of the body only (hemiplegia) or all four limbs may be involved (quadriplegia) with correspondingly greater degrees of handicap. Some forms show marked tremor and unsteadiness (ataxia) whilst others have writhing movements of groups of muscles (athetosis). Depending on the way in which the brain is affected, the development of motor and manipulative skills may be delayed or deviant.

2 The ability to suck, swallow or chew may also be late in developing. Speech in sometimes delayed and may be very indistinct.

3 Some children with cerebral palsy are normally intelligent but others are mentally retarded, which further delays development.

4 Visual defects, particularly squint, and deafness may occur.

5 Fits occur in a proportion of the children.

6 Difficulties in perception become evident as later learning difficulties.

7 Social and emotional problems can arise from isolation, frustration or a rejecting attitude on the part of parents.

Early detection of cerebral palsy enables a full assessment of the degree of disability to be made, and suitable forms of therapy to be planned so as to encourage the child to develop his potential as far as possible. The Spastics Society helps to develop facilities for education, further training and counselling for children with cerebral palsy and aims to promote a greater public awareness of the problem. Local groups enable parents to meet together to discuss mutual experiences and organise social facilities.

Autism

This is a complex condition affecting one child in 5000 and as yet not fully understood. The autistic child appears unable to understand and act upon some of the different stimuli in his environment which ordinarily help development, particularly in its social and language aspects. Autism affects:

1   *Relationships.* The autistic child has great difficulty in making relationships with people, even his mother; he avoids eye contact and does not respond to offers of love and affection.
2   *Speech,* which may not develop at all, or fail to progress beyond the stage of odd words. Speech as a means of communication is lacking.
3   *Play.* Many autistic children prefer toys to social play with other children, but even play with toys is often confined to an obsession with one particular article.
4   *Behaviour* problems are many and varied, ranging from long crying spells and ritualistic behaviour, to temper tantrums and head-banging.

Many autistic children are mentally retarded, but this is not invariably the case.

Unlimited patience is needed to effect even slight changes in behaviour. Parents are advised about ways in which they can encourage eye contact, modify behaviour into more acceptable forms and effect gradual changes of ritual. The National Association for Autistic Children gives information, advice and support for parents.

Muscular dystrophy

There are several forms of muscular dystrophy, of which the most common is the Duchenne type, a hereditary condition occurring in males, caused by the inheritance from the mother of a gene carried on the X (female) chromosome. Duchenne muscular dystrophy is charac- terised by a progressive weakness of the muscles of the legs, later of the arms also, and is usually diagnosed between the age of three to five when difficulty in walking is investigated. There is a gradual deterioration so that by the age of 12 wheelchair life is established and death commonly occurs, before the middle twenties, from respiratory infection or weakening of the cardiac musculature.

The family, understandably, needs a great deal of support and help to enable life to be lived as fully as possible in the face of inevitable early death. Genetic counselling is advised as there is a 50 % risk that another male child will be similarly affected. There is debate as to whether a specific diagnostic blood test should be used in the neonatal period to detect Duchenne muscular dystrophy in boys. Although, as yet, such early diagnosis would do nothing to affect the course and outcome of the disease, it would enable early genetic counselling to be given to the parents who might otherwise produce another affected son before the condition in their first child was realised.

Haemophilia

Haemophilia is a condition occurring only in boys, in which inheritance of a gene from the mother, carried on the X chromosome, causes a total or relative lack of Factor VIII, one of the substances needed for the normal clotting of blood.

In its severe form, there is a risk of spontaneous bleeding into joint cavities, muscles and soft tissues, greatly aggravated by the knocks and bangs which are part of the life of an active young child. Bleeding may also occur from the nose, and in excessive amounts after dental extraction, surgery or injury. In milder forms of haemophilia, the latter risks still remain but spontaneous bleeding is rare.

The bleeding can be stopped by the intravenous injection of a preparation of human Factor VIII. Special haemophilia centres provide facilities for diagnosis, treatment of bleeding as required and at any time, and opportunities for parents to discuss any problems or questions they may wish to raise. Selected haemophiliacs are able to treat themselves at home.

Haemophilia is a rare condition, and is unusual in that its effects are intermittent rather than continuous; the handicap is one of expectancy of possible episodes of interruption of normal life and, in the case of severely affected children, interruption of schooling and restriction of some activities likely to cause injury. They are, however, encouraged to live as normal a life as possible. Parents should be given genetic counselling in order that they appreciate the risks involved in a future pregnancy.

11
Children in Special Circumstances

Many changes have taken place, particularly over the last 30 years, which have affected the structure and stability of the family and the way it functions. It is recognised that changing circumstances, both in society and within individual families, call for a flexible and innovatory approach to the provision of services, so that special as well as common needs can be met. In addition to handicapped children and those in the ethnic minority families, whose needs have already been discussed, the following groups will be considered:

1 Children of working mothers
2 Children in one-parent families
3 Children who are socially disadvantaged

Children of working mothers

Mothers go out to work for a variety of reasons— financial necessity (particularly the single parent), to provide a higher standard of living in the home, or to establish financial independence; others are continuing a vocational career or need the companionship and stimulus that work offers. There is considerable concern that children should not be at any disadvantage because their mother is working, and a great deal depends on the type and duration of the work and the adequacy of substitute care. Children in the early years need as few changes of 'mother substitute' as possible and an environment which is consistently secure and stimulating. Older children require the concern and supervision of a caring adult if the risks of accidents, delinquency and truancy are to be avoided. Conditions of work which include flexibility of working hours, holidays coinciding with those of the school, and leave of absence if the child is ill, all help considerably in arranging satisfactory care. Arrangements may include:

1 *Care in the home by* the father (if interchangeability of role is accepted, flexible working hours permit or where the father is unemployed), by other relatives, granny in particular, or by a nanny or au pair girl.
2 *Care outside the home by* child-minders, day nurseries (either local authority or private), nursery schools or classes.

Many mothers experience some degree of conflict in coming to a decision as to whether or not to go out to work, and the health visitor or social worker is often the person who can help them balance the needs of the child against the expected benefits of work. Those who decide to go out to work may need help to enable them to accept another person's share in the care of their child, and at the same time retain confidence in their own role as a parent. Others who remain at home may benefit from opportunities to enjoy a variety of social contacts, interest activities and stimulation afforded by parent groups and family centres.

Care of children of the working mother

1 In the home by:
   father, relative or nanny
2 Outside the home by:
   child-minder, day nursery or nursery school

Children in one-parent families

It is estimated that one in every eight families is a one-parent family and that one million parents are caring for a million and a half dependent children. A lone parent may be supporting a family because of:

1 Marital breakdown—divorce, separation or desertion, this constitutes the largest proportion of one-parent families.
2 Bereavement.
3 The mother being unmarried. The term 'unmarried mother' covers a whole range of situations from the young girl with little idea of the responsibilities of parenthood, to a woman living in stable cohabitation, who does not strictly come within the concept of one-parent family.

The needs of the one-parent family will vary considerably, depending on individual circumstances and the underlying reasons for absence of a parent. Help is frequently needed to combat financial problems, isolation and difficulties in finding suitable accommodation.

Parental role

A lone parent is normally the sole provider in the family, and is also trying to fulfil the role of two parents in assisting the social and emotional development of the child. There is the additional task of explaining to the child why he differs from the majority of children in having only one parent, whether by reason of divorce, separation, desertion, death or a pregnancy outside marriage. Many one-parent families cope splendidly in the face of great odds, but there is a risk that problems will be intensified by social isolation, by the strain of unrelieved child care (particularly if the child has a severe handicap) and by consequent depression. The health visitor and social worker have a special concern for these families, giving additional support and advice as to services which could offer help. Voluntary organisations such as Gingerbread and Mothers in Action assist one-parent families by initiating self-help parent groups, organising social events, outings and holidays, and providing toy- and clothing-pools. The National Association for One-Parent Families is concerned with safeguarding the interests of these families, offering advice and help to individual parents, and acting as a pressure group where law and social policy are concerned.

Finance

Compared with the majority of two-parent families, the lone parent faces increased financial hardship, particularly in the case of a single, divorced, separated or deserted mother.

Sources of income additional to that obtained through work are:

State benefits The lone parent is entitled to the standard benefits available for all families, or for those whose income is low, with some concessions or extra payment made in view of the special circumstances:

1 *Family income supplement.* The number of working hours needed for qualification is reduced in the case of a lone parent.
2 *Supplementary benefit.* A greater amount of existing income is discounted in deciding the amount allowed. Assessment for this benefit and family income supplement takes into account any maintenance money received.
3 *One-parent benefit:* An extra tax-free weekly amount is granted to a person who has the sole responsibility for bringing up a child or children.
4 *Tax allowances.* Special allowances are granted to the lone parent with a dependent child.

A widowed mother receives a weekly allowance for each child under the age of nineteen years, and a divorced woman with a child is entitled to a child's special allowance if maintenance money ceases on the death of her ex-husband.

Rebates Rate and rent rebates are available for one-parent families, as for all families, when there is difficulty in meeting the full amount.

Court orders
Affiliation order. This order is made in respect of an illegitimate child. The application must be initiated by the mother, either before the birth or within three years of it, and at the time of the application or the birth of the child she must be unmarried, widowed, divorced or separated. The onus is on the mother to substantiate her claim, and blood-tests may be required. If the court (usually the Magistrates' Court) allows the claim, an order is made for a lump sum of money or periodical payments, or both, to be paid by the putative father on behalf of the child. The court has no power to enable any provision to be made for the mother, and affiliation orders usually go only part-way in meeting financial needs. Payments are often irregular and there is difficulty in enforcing them. Private agreement between mother and putative father may be reached outside the court; this usually includes an admission of paternity and is stamped by the court. Many women are reluctant to apply for an affiliation order because of embarrassment, difficulties in proving the claim, or a desire to be independent of the father.

Maintenance order. This is granted by the Divorce Court following proceedings for divorce, nullity or judicial separation. The court takes into account the financial needs and resources of the family when determining the amount of money to be paid.

Accommodation

Financial circumstances usually dictate the type of accommodation which the one-parent family is able to obtain, and this is often less than adequate. Some measure of assistance may be available through:

1 *Local authorities*, making accommodation available suited to the needs of a one-parent family and working in close co-operation with the social services department. The local authority is obliged to find some form of accommodation for homeless families.
2 *Special housing schemes*, offering flatlets or bed-sitting-rooms both in the ante-natal and post-natal periods, at an economic rent and over a reasonable, if not always indefinite, period. Some schemes also offer an advisory service, loan furniture and negotiate with landlords, estate agents and the local authority regarding more permanent accommodation.
3 *Housing advice centres*, which advise on ways in which a family living in a mortgaged house can be protected after marital breakdown.

Work

The lone parent, particularly the mother, often has very limited choice where work is concerned, as much depends on the availability of suitable day care arrangements for the child.

Legal help

Legal help is often needed to enable the lone parent to cope with the complexity of family law:

1 *Legal advice and assistance* is available to people with small incomes, for little or no payment, from some solicitors working from their office or in a legal advice centre. The assistance includes advice, writing letters or getting barristers' opinions, but does not include representation in court proceedings.
2 *Legal aid* is also available, covering the cost of solicitors' fees prior to court appearance and, if necessary, barristers' fees.

The one-parent family needs help in:

1 Maintaining the parental role
2 Finance
3 Accommodation
4 Work
5 Legal help

Children who are socially disadvantaged

This group includes children born into, or growing up in, an environment which could hinder rather than help their growth and development. Some (but not all) children in families where the mother is working, or there is only one parent, are disadvantaged. Social deprivation can also arise in two-parent families in a neighbourhood when:

1 Housing conditions are poor, either in structure, amenities, overcrowding, or lacking facilities for play and social mixing. Interwoven with poor housing is lack of income to ensure adequate nutrition, warmth and clothing (Chapter 1).
2 There are low standards of parental care, stemming from limited intelligence, ignorance about child-rearing or home management.
3 There is maternal depression leading to apathy about the child's welfare and an inability to provide the variety of experiences a child needs for growth and development. Depression sometimes arises secondarily to the poor environmental circumstances or disturbed relationships within the family, but also occurs in mothers where material circumstances are perfectly satisfactory; the feeling of isolation of some young mothers may be a contributory factor.

Social disadvantage has repercussions in many aspects of a child's life and the parents often need special help to enable them to fulfil their responsibilities. The problem of disadvantage is being tackled on many fronts, to enable the cycle of deprivation to be broken:

1   Central and local authorities are aware of the need to review, from time to time, standards of housing and the levels of benefits to which people are entitled. Housing conditions have greatly improved but there still remain areas where rehousing or improvement programmes are awaiting implementation and where private sector accommodation is poor.

2   Concern is expressed that not all families realise the benefits to which they are entitled or how to claim them. Health visitors and social workers should be able to give information in this respect and recent moves to simplify official forms are welcomed; benefits advice centres have been opened in some places.

3   In view of the reluctance of some families to approach the preventive health services, methods of bringing the services to them have been considered. The health visitor, during her home visits and general surveillance of the child, becomes aware of their many problems and, through her knowledge of supporting services and good relationships with the family, may gradually encourage them to take the initiative in health care. The domiciliary family planning service enables mothers to be given contraceptive advice which otherwise they might hesitate to obtain, and mobile clinics can be used for immunisation and general health consultation 'on the doorstep'.

4   Social workers also are frequently involved in the multiple complex problems of disadvantaged families, and not only advise on practical means of assistance, but also try to help parents work through difficult relationships with each other and their children and thus avoid family breakdown (Chapter 9).

5   The education department provides nursery education for children between the ages of two and five years. Nursery teachers are trained in methods which encourage in children the development of physical and intellectual skills, communication and social relationships. This early education can benefit all children, but is specially valuable for those whose home environment could deprive them of full opportunities for development; school health service staff provide health surveillance which might otherwise be difficult to ensure. Many education departments also employ pre-school advisory teachers who visit the home to help parents appreciate ways in which early development can be stimulated, and encourage them to participate in play and learning activities.

6   Local authority day nurseries give priority of admission to children
    who are socially disadvantaged. Family centres provide facilities for
    parents and children to call in for advice, discussion and toy-lending
    facilities. Playgroups also offer a valuable service.

7   Volunteer groups use, for home visiting, mothers from a variety of
    backgrounds and experiences with whom parents can identify,
    discuss problems, and effectively work together.

8   It is essential to develop a co-ordinated approach to home interven-
    tion schemes, both at a policy level and on an individual team basis.

Help for the socially disadvantaged

1   Improved environmental conditions
2   Entitlement to benefit
3   Increased health visiting
4   Social work assistance
5   Educational facilities
6   Day nursery priority
7   Volunteer help
8   Co-ordinated services

Facilities for the care of children outside the home

Day care

Where parents are unable to look after their child for all or part of the
day, and cannot make satisfactory alternative arrangements for care in
the home or with relations, they look for facilities in the community. In
addition to this, professional workers may see the advantage to a child
of spending some part of the day outside the home and away from the
parents, for instance to compensate for social disadvantage or to relieve
situations of stress such as the risk of non-accidental injury.

Day nurseries   Children may be admitted from the age of a few weeks
up to five years, although different authorities vary in their policy to
admit very young babies. The functions of a local authority day nursery
include:

1   Giving material care in the form of shelter, food, warmth and, at
    times, clothing. Nurseries are open for most of the year from around
    8.0 a.m. until 6.0 p.m.

2 Providing health care. The nursery also affords excellent opportunities for surveillance of health and development, and many districts make arrangements for regular visits by a health visitor and clinical medical officer. A proportion of children attending day nurseries have not been immunised and arrangements can be made for this to be done. Health education, appropriate to the age of the child, can be commenced in areas such as dental health and safety.

3 An educational role in encouraging the development of social independence in feeding, toilet training and dressing. A wide range of toys and play facilities provide stimulus to general development.

4 Work with families. More and more nurseries are recognising this contribution to parent education and support, in trying to build up the relationship between child and parents. Parents are welcomed for whole or part of the day, encouraged to participate in activities and offered opportunities for informal discussion with staff or amongst themselves.

5 Facilities for older children. In some instances nurseries are combined with facilities for supervision of older children after school hours until such time as parents are able to resume their care.

The nurseries are staffed by qualified nursery nurses in ratios appropriate to the number and age of the children. There is local variation as to whether or not a fee is chargeable; if there is a charge, the amount usually varies according to the need and the family income.

Private day nurseries, whether run by charitable organisations or individuals, are encouraged to adopt standards of care comparable to those run by the local authorities. In order to ensure conditions satisfactory for the health, welfare and safety of children, there is a legal obligation that private nurseries register with the social services department, and they must conform to conditions relating to suitability of premises and staff laid down in the Nurseries and Child-Minders Acts. Private nurseries determine their own fees and hours of service.

Child-minders The legal definition of a child-minder is a person other than a relative who looks after a child under the age of five years in the minder's home for more than two hours a day for reward in money or in kind. All child-minders are required by law to register with the social services department, and conditions similar to those required for private day nurseries must be met. Child-minders are free to charge what they wish for their services, although to some extent this is influenced by the estimated ability of the parent to pay. Some local authorities have schemes whereby needy parents are subsidised to help them place their child with a satisfactory minder. Health visitors are usually informed by the social services department when a child is placed with a minder, as it is important that (with the parents' permission) surveillance of health is continued as if the child were at home.

Much concern is felt about child-minders who are operating illegally by failing to register their practice, and who are thus difficult to trace. Because of their low fees, such minders tend to be used by lone parents, those from ethnic minority groups, or from socially disadvantaged homes. The minder's home itself is often unsatisfactory, too many children are received, there are few play facilities and little stimulation of any kind. Far from providing an opportunity for an already disadvantaged child to benefit from alternative care, they perpetuate the pattern of disadvantages. It has been suggested that positive inducements to register should be offered, such as financial help to provide equipment and toys, and a recognised course of training which some authorities already organise. Such courses include tuition on the needs of young children, and also emphasise the potential value of child-minders' care in the important early years of life, thus giving them a sense of status within the sphere of pre-school provisions. Some social services departments employ day foster-parents (child-minders who are paid a salary by the department) and an extension of this system could result in generally higher standards of care.

Nursery school   As well as providing opportunity for learning, the nursery school also affords a secure environment for the child. For many mothers working full-time, however, nursery schools are of limited value where day care is concerned because of their short hours and observance of school holidays. Provisions which combine the facilities of full day nursery care and nursery class education are of great value.

Day care facilities

1   Day nursery
2   Child-minder
3   Nursery school, to a limited extent

Full care facilities

It is recognised that separation of a child from home and parents is a very serious step and should only be taken when other measures prove to be inadequate or the child's well-being is jeopardised. Full care may be needed for some children, either on a temporary or permanent basis, when supporting day-time services are insufficient to meet needs.

Private arrangements   Many parents make private arrangements with relations or friends, particularly for short periods of time, or use the services of private foster-parents; this may be from choice or because their needs do not fall within the categories for which local authority care services are available. Private fostering is subject to legal requirements designed to protect the child from poor standards of care.

Local authority care   The local authority has a responsibility to provide a child care service which is *offered* to families (i.e. voluntary care) where a specific need is indicated:

1   When one or both parents are mentally or physically ill, or there are any other circumstances which cause them to be unable to provide proper care for the child. Short-term illness of a parent is the most common reason for reception into care.
2   When a child has no parent or guardian, or has been abandoned.
3   When it would seem to be in the best interests of the child that he is away from his parents.

Reception into voluntary care is dependent on the parents' consent, and parents have the right to take back their child at any time within a period of six months. When a child has been continuously in care for six months or longer, parents must give 28 days' notice of their intention to reclaim their child. This gives time for a gradual re-introduction of the child back into the family or, when return is not considered to be in the best interests of the child, it allows the local authority to prepare for further action. When circumstances seem permanent enough to indicate that parental care can never be satisfactorily resumed (such as death of both parents, permanent disability or a mode of life which makes rehabilitation unlikely) the local authority may take over the parental rights as well as responsibility. Once this has been assumed, parents lose their right to reclaim the child unless, and until, the local authority thinks fit, or the court gives judgement in the parents' favour. When refusal of voluntary care seriously threatens the child's well-being, legal enforcement may be sought (Chapter 11).

Arrangements for care

When the local authority takes a child into care, the aim is to provide the type of substitute care which is most suitable for an individual child:

Fostering (or boarding-out)   The social services department must follow legal regulations in the selection of foster-parents in that they consider the applicants to be appropriate people with a home suitable for the care of a child. Efforts are made to place a child with foster-parents most suitable for his individual needs, particularly if the placement is anticipated to be long-term (more than eight weeks). Foster-parents are paid by the local authority, and they can include relations of the child. A pre-placement medical examination of the child is required and regular health examinations continue at least every six months in a child under the age of two, every year in older children. The social worker plays an important part in the initial placement, in the support of the foster-parents, and regular supervision of the child's progress.

Whether foster-parents are acting in a private capacity or are paid by the local authority, their role demands not only the ability to provide material comfort, but an understanding of the child's psychological needs and the ability to appreciate the parents' rights, even though the foster-parents have assumed parental responsibility.

Community homes   The placement of a child in a community home is an alternative to individual fostering. A community home may be a residential nursery or a family group home in which eight or ten children of different ages are cared for by a married couple acting as substitute parents. The homes aim to provide a family life in the community; the children attend the local school and participate in neighbourhood activities. Other community homes are run by voluntary organisations with varying degrees of involvement of the local authority regarding financial help and staffing. All community' homes are subject to legal regulations.

Full care arrangements

1   Private fostering or individual home
2   Local authority care:
    Foster home
    Community home

Adoption

Adoption is the means by which a child is given a permanent new home when his own family is unable or unwilling to care for him. The new parents are prepared to assume all parental rights and responsibilities, and because adoption is irrevocable, it is essential that great care is taken to ensure it is in the best interests of the child and that it will provide the love, security and material care that the child needs. Decisions about adoption are made after detailed consideration by qualified social workers and other experienced people associated with an adoption agency; third party and private adoptions are no longer legal. The decision must then be legalised by a court order (usually the County Court).

Adoption and the law   The process of adoption is governed by legal requirements set out in the Adoption Act (1958) with amendments made in The Children Act (1975). The law makes various stipulations:

The adopters, in every instance, must be over the age of 21 years. No maximum age limit is laid down in law, but individual adoption agencies may impose their own upper age limits. Both married and single people are eligible to adopt, but apart from a single mother or relative adopting the child, it is probable that most adoption agencies would choose to place a child in the traditional two-parent family.

The child must be under the age of 18 years, and have never been married.

Consent for adoption. Before an adoption order is made the Court must be satisfied that the necessary consents have been made. In the case of a single mother her consent is sufficient, but when a married couple place their child for adoption the consent of both parents is needed. Consent may be waived if the parents cannot be found, if the child is neglected, or if there has been persistent or serious ill-treatment of the child to the extent that his rehabilitation into the family is unlikely. The consent is not legally valid until six weeks after the birth and can be withdrawn at any time before the adoption order is made.

The adoption process. The child must have lived with the adopting parents for a continuous period of three months (not counting the first six weeks of life) before an adoption order can be made. This period is to allow the adopting parents and the child time to get used to each other and to feel confident that the placement is the right one for them. A social worker visits the family during this period, and a 'guardian *ad litem*' is appointed (usually a probation officer or a social worker from a different agency) to present an independent report to the court on the adopters, the child and the opinion of the professional worker involved with the family.

The court order. When the court is satisfied that the adoption is in the best interests of the child, that both the natural and adopting parents understand its implications, and the necessary consents have been given, the order can then be made, transferring all the parental rights and responsibilities to the adopting parents. The adoption is recorded in the Adopted Children's Register and information linking the new name with the original birth registration is kept by the Registrar General as a confidential record. A new birth certificate is made out in the child's adopted name.

Information on origins. Since 1976, adopted people over the age of 18 have the right to be given information about their birth origins. Those adopted before the end of 1975 are required to see a specially appointed counsellor before any information can be given; a person adopted after this date is offered the opportunity for counselling if he wishes, but otherwise may obtain the information directly from the Registrar General or the local authority in which he lives. The purpose of counselling is to help the adopted person understand adoption and its procedures, and some of the possibly distressful effects of enquiries if pursued to the limit. The counsellor then gives information from the adoption order, which includes the person's original name and that of the parents, and the applicant can, if he wishes, obtain a copy of the original birth registration. The right to information was introduced because it was felt that some adopted people, particularly if they received little information from their adopting parents, have a need to know something of their origin in order to establish their identity as a person.

The law on adoption

1 Approved agency adoptions only
2 Stipulations about adopters and the child
3 Legal consent
4 The three months' period
5 The court order
6 Information on origins

The adoption agency An adoption agency may form part of the local authority social services department or be a charitable agency approved by the Department of Health. The agency receives applications from prospective adopters and from a mother, or parents, wishing to place their child for adoption. Before couples are accepted as adopting parents, several interviews have taken place with experienced social workers working with the agency. Reasons for wishing to adopt a child are discussed, together with their views on the needs of children, attitudes to telling the child about adoption, feelings towards parents who place their child for adoption, and their expectations of an adopted child. An opinion is formed on the couple's ability to provide a home which is adequate (but not necessarily luxurious) in a material sense, but which must certainly be loving, secure and stimulating. Discussions also take place with the natural mother; many babies placed for adoption are those born to single women. Ideally, this should take place during the ante-natal period, as the essential purpose is to help the mother come to a carefully considered decision about the future of her baby, made in the light of her own circumstances, a knowledge of the options open to her, and an understanding of the implications both of keeping and relinquishing the baby. Unhurried counselling often succeeds in preventing last-minute uncertainty and withdrawal of consent. In recent years, there has been a trend towards considering adoption for older children who may have been in local authority care for some time. Parental consent is still necessary unless there are valid grounds for dispensing with it and, where adopting parents are concerned, there is the need to assess their ability to deal with children who may already be disturbed because of their past experiences.

The medical aspects of adoption   The court insists on medical reports on parents and child before arriving at a decision on adoption. The adoption agency is advised by an experienced doctor with a special interest in adoption work, who interprets the significance of medical findings in the light of the proposed adoption procedures.

The adopting parents. The main consideration is not just their good health at the time of examination, but a reasonable assumption that they will remain healthy over the length of time an adopted child needs their care. Clearly, it is not possible to forecast every eventuality in the coming years, but the medical history and clinical examination, together with any specialist reports considered necessary, help the medical adviser to give his judgement.

The child. A child under consideration for adoption has a pre-placement medical assessment and a further one shortly before the application is heard in court.

The purpose of the pre-placement medical assessment is to be able to give the prospective adopters a picture of the child's health, development and family background and, as far as possible, an idea of future progress. Some couples express a wish for a 'normal' child and, whilst the possibility of untoward happenings cannot be excluded, it is possible in many instances to say that development is normal for the child's age and that there is nothing at the time of examination to suggest that it will not continue to be so. In a few instances there may be obvious anomalies of development, such as a congenital heart lesion or Down's syndrome; this does not necessarily mean that this child cannot be adopted, as some applicants are willing to take a child with special needs. It is essential that, before agreeing to take such a child, the applicants fully understand the nature of the disability, any treatment indicated, the extent to which it is anticipated that this will be effective, and how future development (both short- and long-term) is likely to be affected. If there is doubt about future progress of any child opinion can be deferred if a future examination is likely to resolve the issue one way or the other, or the baby can be placed with adopters who are able to tolerate the doubt, whatever its outcome. It is most important that the child's assessment should be carried out by a skilled and experienced doctor to prevent the tragedy of parents adopting a child in the expectation of normality when the signs of abnormality were present at the time of examination, or of a child being deprived of adoption because the real significance of doubtful findings was not appreciated.

The decision   The agency adoption committee includes social workers and other professional people; they discuss all the reports relating to prospective adopters and to children put forward for adoption, together with any relevant references, and a decision is made on acceptance or rejection. The committee does not necessarily decide that a particular couple adopt a particular baby; this is left to the judgement of the social workers most involved with individual applications. The baby may be placed with the prospective adopters directly from the maternity unit, or may spend six weeks or longer in foster care prior to placement; where possible, placement is made at an early age to enable parent/child attachment to develop fully.

After placement   If this is the adopting parents' first experience of the care of a child, an opportunity should be given in the pre-placement period for them to participate in health education groups on the practical aspects of child care, patterns of development, and the needs of children. The health visitor is notified of a placement and she will offer her services to the family with recognition of the needs of adopting parents for reassurance and encouragement, particularly during the months before the order is made. The question of telling the child that he is adopted is discussed with the parents by the social worker during the preliminary interviews, but once the adoption order has been made, the social worker withdraws from the scene and the mother may turn to the health visitor for help in the practicality of 'telling'.

The medical aspects of adoption

1   Medical certificates needed by court
2   The adopting parents—fitness to care for a child
3   The child—an assessment of present health and development and future outlook
4   The support for adopting parents

The future

Much help in the form of home services, day facilities and full-time care is available for children in families where parents are unable to draw on their own resources in providing satisfactory care. Future developments, not only in ensuring the adequacy of alternative sources of care, but in ensuring that those providing it (child-minders and foster-parents) have knowledge of the special needs of these children and adequate support to enable them to give the quality of care which will overcome disadvantage and ensure a child's future well-being.

12

Non-accidental Injury

The place and status of children in western society has changed gradually over the years. The majority of children today are no longer regarded as mini-adults or as part of the parents' goods and chattels, but rather as people in their own right, with needs of their own to be met. Harsh treatment of children by parents which was formerly tolerated as being appropriate, and at times even encouraged 'for their own good', is now regarded in a totally different light, and with this change has emerged a focusing of concern on non-accidental injury and the circumstances in which it arises.

Non-accidental injury is defined as a clinical condition in children who have received physical abuse, generally from a parent or other person who has care of them. It forms part of a wide spectrum of conditions which include:

1 Physical injury.
2 Emotional trauma, which is often inextricably bound up with physical cruelty, but may exist as an entity in itself and result in behaviour problems, poor emotional adjustment and growth failure (Chapter 4).
3 Acts of omission, neglect and deprivation, the boundaries of which merge imperceptibly into physical and emotional injury, and which are equivalent to cruelty because the normal needs of the child are not being met.
4 Sexual abuse within the family, which is causing increasing concern.

Prevention of non-accidental injury

Most parents are able to provide conditions in which their children can develop and fulfil their potential, but some parents subject them to neglect and abuse. Although non-accidental injury is a clinical entity, it is also a symptom of underlying disruptive forces and its prevention must be considered in the context of family relationships and the internal and external resources which are available to help parents fulfil their role successfully. Research based on known cases of child abuse has given considerable insight into the under-lying factors which operate.

Family structure

The parents are often very young and have had two or three children in rapid succession; the pregnancy is frequently pre- or extra-marital and unplanned. The parents are unable to cope with the needs of several small children, and a premature baby, handicapped or hyperactive child is particularly vulnerable by reason of the increased demands on parental care and energy. Young children under the age of three appear to be at greatest risk of non-accidental injury, although it does occur in older age groups too.

Parental experience

The parents' own experiences in childhood are frequently those of rejection and ill-treatment from their own parents. This not only perpetuates a model of child-rearing which incorporates violence, but may also have affected the parents' personality so much that they cannot accept and fulfil satisfactorily the role of parenthood.

Parents often have little understanding of the stages of normal development and have unrealistic expectations of the child's achievement, behaviour and responses of love and affection towards them. The stages of 'messy' feeding, incomplete bladder control and negativism through which every child passes are interpreted as acts of disobedience needing punishment. Episodes such as an irritable crying baby or sleep and feeding problems present extra stress and may be seen by the parents as reflections on their capability or as the child being deliberately difficult.

There may be additional factors in one or both parents such as mental illness, subnormality, criminal tendencies and problems with alcohol.

Social stresses

Many families in which non-accidental injury occurs belong to social classes four and five, and are living in conditions of poor housing, low income and insecurity, which add to their inherent difficulties of child-rearing. These factors in themselves do not cause non-accidental injury; many families in such circumstances provide loving care for their children and, conversely, child abuse can occur in children from homes where material conditions are good.

Social isolation is common; the parents lack the support of their own families, either by choice, or because of geographical isolation. Their generally hostile attitude prevents them from making close friends or participating in neighbourhood activities.

Families 'at risk'

1 Family structure:
     Young parents with a large family
     Young children, particularly if premature or handicapped.
2 The parents:
     Poor past experience
     Lack of knowledge of children's needs
     Personality traits
3 Social stresses:
     Poverty
     Isolation

Primary prevention of non-accidental injury depends on:

1 Professional workers being aware of a potentially dangerous situation created by family circumstances.
2 Ways being found to give parents help and support in building up their nurturing capacity and relieving stress.

The ante-natal period

Unhurried discussion in the ante-natal period can uncover signs anticipating possible difficulty in establishing a good mother/child relationship. The pregnancy may be unplanned and unwanted, continuing after a request for abortion has been refused; it is important that counselling should continue to help the mother work through her feelings of resentment and rejection. Practical advice regarding sources of possible financial support and improved housing is offered, and the content of parent-craft classes should be such as to convey a realistic picture of infant care and development.

At birth

The mother's first reactions to her baby give indication of her attitude towards him. The importance is recognised of immediate skin-to-skin contact of mother and baby in helping to establish a close, warm relationship (bonding). Throughout the immediate post-natal period there should be frequent opportunities for the mother to hold, handle and cuddle her baby. When intensive care is needed for the newborn baby, arrangements are made to promote bonding as far as is possible

(Chapter 3). In some maternity units, special facilities are provided for those mothers thought to need help in developing their mothering capacity.

At home

1 Health visitors and community midwives are aware of 'risk factors' in the families they visit, and recognise the special need for supportive care, particularly in episodes of feeding difficulties or a crying baby. Increased frequency of visiting, time spent in listening to the parents and explanations of the stages of development and responses of children may uncover strengths in the family on which to build. Referral to the domiciliary family planning service and to other agencies may be indicated. The social worker gives more intensive casework and organises the provision of supporting facilities. Psychiatric help may be needed, or a consultation with a paediatrician regarding the child's general progress.

2 Parents frequently need some reassurance that out-of-hours advice and help is available at times when frustration mounts. Some districts provide this as part of the health visiting or midwifery service; in others, voluntary bodies such as the National Society for the Prevention of Cruelty to Children (NSPCC) respond to cries for help, and other groups such as Parent Lifeline offer a telephone contact, usually a mother herself, to whom parents can express their anxieties and frustrations.

3 All parents, at times, feel the need for a short period of relief from child care, and for families where there is a risk of non-accidental injury, this relief is even more important. Help can be provided through:

(a) Playgroups.
(b) Mother and toddler groups.
(c) Day nursery or nursery class.
(d) Volunteers who will 'baby-sit' or, from time to time, have care of the child for two or three hours.

Such facilities relieve social isolation, provide a means by which understanding of normal development can be learned, and act as checks on unacceptable behaviour towards the child.

4 It is important to explore means by which housing and financial difficulties may be resolved (Chapter 1).

5 The National Society for the Prevention of Cruelty to Children is an important voluntary body which aims to provide immediate help for children in need, particularly those who are neglected or at risk of

abuse. A 24-hour service is provided; practical help is organised and the workers also concentrate in the fostering of a good relationship between parent and child. Special units are set up in some places providing a round-the-clock relief service which offers psychological and psychiatric assessment for parent and child. The NSPCC has also undertaken many research studies into non-accidental injury.

6 Workers in many agencies are involved in the care of the 'at risk' family, and it is important that a co-ordinated approach to care be made, both in individual families and on a broad policy basis. Each district has set up a review committee on which are represented the health services, social services and education departments, the police and probation services and the NSPCC. The function of the review committee is:

(a) To monitor the incidence of known and suspected cases of non-accidental injury.
(b) To encourage co-ordination of services and joint consultation.
(c) To formulate policies on the procedure to be followed in cases of confirmed or suspected non-accidental injury.
(d) To maintain a central register of known and suspected cases, and also of families considered to be 'at risk'. The register is maintained by the social services department, health authority or NSPCC, is reviewed at regular intervals and can be consulted by professional workers who need information on individual families with whom they come into contact.

Prevention of non-accidental injury

1 Help and support for families at risk, from midwife, health visitor, social workers
2 Out of hours service
3 Relief of social isolation
4 Help with finance and housing
5 The work of the NSPCC
6 Co-ordination of care

The injured child

It is important that professional staff working in the community and in hospital should be aware of the possibility that injury to a child may be deliberate, particularly when family circumstances are known to place the child at risk. Accidents in childhood are common, and there is a need for balance so that on, the one hand, non-accidental injury is not missed and, on the other, undue suspicion is avoided which could cause mistrust to the extent that some parents would be reluctant to seek help. Non-accidental injury is suspected when:

1 There is delay in seeking advice for conditions which the majority of parents would feel merit speedy attention.
2 There is a history of repeated injuries.
3 The parents' account casts doubt on the way in which the injury is reported to have been caused; the explanation may be inadequate or outside the limits of probability in view of the child's stage of development.
4 The injury is not of a type usually associated with purely accidental happenings.
5 The parents show a degree of concern or unconcern out of proportion to the seriousness of the injury.

Start to wonder when there are:

1 Delays in seeking advice
2 Repeated injuries
3 Unsatisfactory explanations
4 Atypical injuries
5 Abnormal parental attitudes

Types of injury

Bruises Bruising is a common feature of accidental injury, but deliberate action is suspected when they are found on the face and around the mouth, and when there are multiple bruises of different ages as indicated by the colour changes. Finger mark bruises may be seen, and human bites show as open-ended bruises.

Bone injuries Fractures of the skull, ribs and long bones, and joint injuries may be found. Suspicion is aroused by fractures with marked displacement in the long bones, in contrast to the greenstick fracture commonly seen as the result of accidental injury in young children. X-rays may show old fractures in different stages of healing.

Bleeding This may occur:
1 From the mouth as a result of a torn frenulum due to forcible thrusting of the teat into the mouth, or to gum or teeth injury from direct blows.

2   As a subdural haematoma resulting from blows to the head or violent shaking. This gives rise to persistent vomiting and, in a young baby, to an abnormal increase in head circumference.
3   As ocular haemorrhages from violent shaking; these are seen on ophthalmoscopic examination.
4   In the abdomen from a ruptured liver or spleen due to blows on the abdomen.

Burns and scalds   These present characteristic appearances depending on the means by which the injury was inflicted. Cigarette burns show as discrete small circular lesions and indicate a degree of premeditation.

Poisoning   Deliberate overdosage of drugs may be a feature of non-accidental injury.

Signs of severe neglect   These include unexplained failure to thrive, and severe nappy-rash (although this can occur in the absence of neglect).

Types of injury

1   Bruises
2   Bone injuries
3   Bleeding
4   Burns and scalds
5   Poisoning
6   Severe neglect

If non-accidental injury is suspected it is important to examine the whole child, including X-ray of the skull, thorax and limbs, and to record accurately the full extent of the injuries.

Procedure in cases of suspected non-accidental injury

In addition to the medical diagnosis and treatment of the injury, the aims of the management are:

1   To safeguard the child from further injury, both in the immediate and long-term future.
2   Where possible, to work towards long-term improvement of the family situation.

Safeguarding the child

A place of safety   If it is felt that the child is at risk of further injury by allowing him to remain at home, he is safeguarded by removal to a place of safety, which is usually a hospital ward, or may be a foster home or residential home. Most parents will consent to hospital admission, particularly if the approach is made in a non-accusatory way and by advising that investigation of the child's condition is necessary. This is a wise procedure in any case to ensure a correct diagnosis and exclude pathological conditions such as bleeding disorders or fragilitas ossium (brittle bones).

If the parents refuse to allow the child to be admitted, a *place of safety order* may be sought. This order is given by a magistrate after hearing an application in person from the social services department or the NSPCC. The application can be made at any time, day or night, and the order remains in force for 28 days, during which time the parents cannot remove the child unless the order is revoked.

The case conference   The holding of the child in a place of safety allows time for a case conference to be called, the central register to be consulted and for further investigations to be made into the total circumstances surrounding the happening. The case conference is usually held as soon as possible after admission of the child but, in any case, before he is discharged. It includes all professional workers involved with the family or having relevant information to contribute. The aim of the conference is to come to a decision regarding the future of the child after the 28 day period of the place of safety order has elapsed and to nominate a key worker who will undertake intensive work with the family and act as a co-ordinator of care. The police are generally invited to a case conference, but they retain the right to decide regarding prosecution.

Options for future care   The case conference may decide that there is insufficient evidence to warrant taking the case to a court, and the child is allowed to return home under voluntary supervision of the key worker. Otherwise the case is taken to the juvenile court with a recommendation that legal protection is advisable; this may be in the form of:

1   *A care order*, by which the child is removed from the damaging environment of his own home and placed with foster parents or a community home. The local authority assumes all parental responsibilities in relation to the child. The order can remain in force until the child is 18 years old, and the parents cannot remove the child from care unless the order is cancelled. The local authority or the parents may make an application for the order to be terminated, and in the latter case the court will make a decision in the light of the parents' evidence and that of professional workers involved with the child and family.

2 *A supervision order*, which allows the child to return home on condition that the parents accept for a maximum period of three years, supervision from a social worker or probation officer. The term 'supervision' is interpreted to include constructive work with the parents but if, in spite of this, the child appears to be in renewed danger, a care order is sought.

Work with parents

When a child is allowed to remain at home under voluntary or legal supervision, every effort is made to build up a more satisfactory relationship between parents and child, and to alleviate social stresses so that the risk of non-accidental injury recedes. The decision to remove a child from the care of his parents is a serious one, and is taken only when this appears to be in the best interests of the child. Although a care order may remain in force until the child is 18 years old, consideration is always given to the possibility of return home should conditions improve to the extent that it would be safe for him to do so. Continuing work with the parents is undertaken by a social worker or probation officer; visiting of the child is encouraged if rehabilitation within the family appears a possibility. Even whilst the care order is operative, the child may be allowed home for a trial period after full consultation with other workers involved with the family and under close supervision. Other children in the family, if remaining at home, also need very careful supervision and, should another pregnancy occur, inter-professional consultation should take place regarding plans for the baby's future.

Management of non-accidental injury

1 Treat the injuries
2 Remove the child to a place of safety
3 The case conference
4 Plans for the child's future
5 Work with parents

A great deal has already been achieved in the identification of families in which non-accidental injury of children is a possibility. Different preventive and therapeutic approaches are being tried so as to develop strengths within the family, enabling them to provide adequately for their children. Both for children at risk and those who, tragically, have already suffered injury at the hands of their parents, the task lies not only in safeguarding them in the present, but also in trying to overcome the effects of their early experiences so as to prevent perpetuation of the problem through the next generation. The ramifications of non-accidental injury extend into the society in which families live. Improvements in material conditions are needed to help many families function adequately; but beyond this is the need to tackle wider problems in the environment of children, including present-day attitudes to family life and the intrusion of violence in its many forms.

13

Bereavement in the Family

Many conditions which formerly caused death in children are now preventable and curable, and in contrast to life a hundred years ago, when death in young children was accepted as a possibility, the general expectation today is that a child will survive into healthy adulthood. This makes it all the more devastating when death does occur, whether due to an incurable malignancy, a congenital abnormality or, even more so, when it happens in an apparently healthy child as a result of accident or 'cot death'. Most families have relatives or friends to whom they can turn for comfort and who will sustain them during their period of mourning. The role of the health professional worker is also an important one in helping bereaved parents and children to work through the period of distress and consolidate their life as a family.

Sharing of grief

Many families are helped when they are able to feel that professional workers understand the depths of their loss and share in their grief because they have also shared in the life and care of the child. Sharing of grief also involves the understanding of parents' feelings in cases of still-birth and neo-natal death where independent life has not been established, or is of short duration. Most parents perceive life as starting during pregnancy, and perinatal death represents a loss to them which is difficult to bear because ways in which they would ordinarily have come to know their baby as part of the family have been so limited. Help can be given during the immediate post-natal period by a sensitive approach to individual needs, and by offering parents the opportunity to see, touch and hold their dead baby so that he becomes a real person to them. It is important that the general practitioner and health visitor get early information about the death of a child of any age, to enable them to make contact with the family. The initial visit may be a brief one to express sympathy, but it carries with it the assurance of concern and of help and support in the future.

Working through grief

In the days and weeks that follow the death of a child, many parents feel the need of someone apart from the family, with a knowledge of child health, who has the time, perhaps on repeated occasions, to listen with understanding and compassion to their questions, and the outpourings of their conscious feelings of sorrow, guilt and anger. Counsellors are able to understand and interpret the many ways through which grief is revealed, and can accept hostile expressions of resentment as being not necessarily directed against themselves personally, but rather against the services they represent, which in the parents' eyes were not able to save their child. There may be at times, indeed, valid criticisms of a service, which are important to recognise and use in ways which will improve the delivery of health care. The general practitioner, family health visitor and, sometimes, the social worker are often able to give ongoing counselling, building on their existing relationship with the family; sometimes a specialist health visitor will have been closely involved, over a period of time, in the care of a child with a terminal illness, and will continue her support after death.

Information about the cause of death

Many parents find discussion with a consultant paediatrician or paediatric pathologist helpful in enabling them to understand more clearly the reasons for death occurring, or when this is inexplicable (as in some cases of 'cot deaths') to accept the limitations of medical knowledge and the assurance that their own management of the child and that of health workers was not at fault. Advice may also be given about the need for genetic counselling and arrangements in the event of a future pregnancy. Information shared between hospital and community health staff enables a reinforcement of support to be given when, as so often happens, repeated explanation and reassurance are sought by the parents.

Practical help

Advice and help in practicalities, given in a sensitive way, also serve as expressions of concern and often open the way for ongoing counselling to take place.

Registration procedures

The death must be registered with the local registrar within five days of the event occurring. A still-birth must also be registered and, although the statutory period allowed is 42 days, early registration enables arrangements for burial to proceed. In either case, the certificate from the registrar enables the formalities for burial or cremation to be completed and, in the case of a death (but not a still-birth), application for the death grant to be made. The death grant is a sum of money, dependent on insurance contributions, which varies in amount with the age of the person. A parent receiving supplementary benefit may also be granted money to help with essential funeral expenses.

Funeral procedures

The District Health Authority can, if the parents so wish, arrange a funeral free of charge for a still-born baby, whether born in hospital or at home. The parents are relieved of the necessity to make arrangements but it is important they are informed when and where the burial will take place. Apart from this and local provision whereby some hospital authorities make arrangements for the burial of a baby dying in the early neonatal period, the parents make private arrangements for burial or cremation. The cost of a private funeral varies a great deal, but is often high enough to cause financial embarrassment to young couples. It is probable that the amount of the death grant will be increased in the future.

Medical and nursing help

The family doctor, health visitor and community midwife are able to discuss and give advice on situations commonly associated with loss of a child, such as:

1 Sleep problems and other physical symptoms arising out of grief.
2 Suppression of lactation.
3 The question of another pregnancy and at what stage this is to be contemplated. It is thought wiser to help parents move through their period of mourning towards an individual decision regarding the conception of another child, who will be valued for himself and not as a replacement for the dead child.
4 Contraceptive advice where appropriate.
5 The need for psychiatric help.

Other help

Health staff are in a position to suggest other agencies which might help bereaved parents. The social services department offers skilled social work help in resolving family difficulties which may become accentuated following the loss of a child. Voluntary associations such as the Foundation for the Study of Infant Deaths and the Still-Birth Association encourage the formation of local support groups through which parents may find help and comfort by sharing their mutual problems with other parents.

Bereavement counselling

1 Sharing of grief
2 Working through grief
3 Factual information about the cause of death
4 Practical help
5 Mobilisation of helping agencies

Help for bereaved children

Children may suffer bereavement by loss of a parent or a sibling, and it is important that their needs are not overlooked. Much depends on the age of the child as to his understanding of death, particularly its finality, which is probably not appreciated realistically until the age of ten or eleven. All children, however, feel loss by reason of separation and need comfort and counselling to help them come to terms with their grief and feelings of anger and resentment. They do not always react in an adult way—they may show apparent unconcern which masks their deeper distress and fear that they, too, or the other parent may also disappear; questions are not always asked and so fantasies and feelings of guilt that the situation is somehow their fault could remain unresolved. A child is helped by:

1 Simple truthful explanation within his capacity to understand.
2 Encouragement to express his feelings and to ask questions; in younger children observation of play often gives some indication.
3 Recognition of some of the indirect expressions of grief and insecurity in physical symptoms (loss of appetite, sleep disturbance and enuresis), emotional and behavioural difficulties. Referral for paediatric advice or to the child psychological service may be indicated.
4 Gradual introduction in the course of everyday life to the concept of the finiteness of existence as shown in nature, the death of a pet, or distant relative.

Support and help for the parent enables them in their turn to help the child. It is sometimes valuable to involve a professional worker such as a health visitor or teacher who is aware of the child's needs and, because she is less emotionally involved than the parent, can offer support which is acceptable and effective. An experienced counsellor may be needed to help the adolescent through the crisis of losing of a parent at a time when areas of personal identity and relationships are being explored. 'Cruse' (The National Organisation for the Widowed and their Children) offers a counselling service and has a special concern to help the bereaved parent in aspects of child management.

Help for the child

1   Truthful explanations
2   Expression of feelings
3   Recognition of signs of hidden grief and insecurity
4   Health education
5   A special counsellor

14
The Future

Great changes have taken place over the past thirty years or so in the whole field of health and welfare of children and their families. Many of these changes have their roots in the distant past, particularly in the reforms of the nineteenth century, but in recent decades they have gained momentum. The United Nations' 'Declaration of the Rights of the Child' confronts us with one of the most fundamental issues—the acknowledgment that the child has rights, amongst them the right to survive, to grow up in an atmosphere of affection and security, to be given opportunities and facilities to enable him to develop in a healthy and normal manner, to enjoy the benefits of social security, including adequate nutrition, housing, recreation and medical care. These are rights which services of the future, as well as of today, are being challenged to meet (Fig. 14.1).

The majority of children in this country can now expect a great deal of life where health is concerned. The development of preventive and curative health services has promoted the child's right not only to

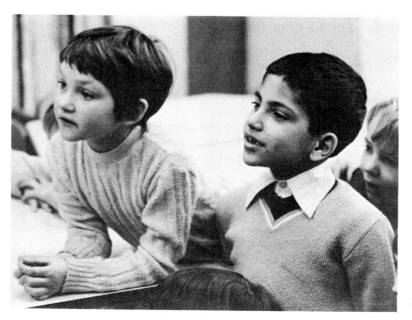

Fig. 14.1 Fit for the future. *Colin New*

survive, but to do so with good quality of life. There remain, however, the special needs of the ethnic minority groups, the disadvantaged families, children at risk of non-accidental injury, the handicapped child, and children in care. There is the contrast of poverty for some and plenty for others, and the paradox of services being there and not being used. The design of services for the future will continue to make provision for special as well as general needs, and will recognise the threats to health that may arise because of changes in the social environment, particularly job insecurity.

Child health of the future can be promoted by three major influences—the parents, planners and providers, and society.

The parents

Recent years have seen a tremendous upsurge of enthusiasm to promote opportunities for parents to learn more about child health and development, and to help them in their task of parenting. There is a continued need to develop a variety of approaches, particularly for those parents who would not of their own initiative come forward to use the services. The aim should be to give help in a way which, because it is acceptable, will carry reassurance, develop confidence and enable them to enjoy their children. Particularly important is the need to help them recognise, from amongst the common characteristics of all children, the individuality of their own child and to tailor general principles to the child's needs so as to give a 'bespoke' rather than 'off the peg' upbringing.

Planners and providers

There has been a welcome recognition of the importance of social elements in environmental planning, particularly in the design of housing and facilities for play, but the immense complexity of poor conditions, particularly in inner city areas, has still to be resolved. Where health services are concerned, there is a continued need to examine services and their uptake, to identify real or potential barriers preventing their use, and to provide a range of services which is flexible enough to meet the changing requirements of children in whatever circumstances they are living—at home, in hospital or in care, in rural communities or large cities.

Changes stemming from the 1982 health service reorganisation will hopefully encourage more integration of hospital and community services, thus enabling a greater degree of co-ordinated care to be given because the total circumstances of the child's life and that of his family are fully appreciated. There is an urgent need to ensure that the planning of child health services lies in the hands of people who, in practice as well as in theory, are fully conversant with the principles of child health. It is equally urgent to implement a recognised programme of training to develop the special skills and contribution of the clinical medical officers who, together with the general practitioners and health visitors, are in closest contact with the child and parents in matters of community health care.

Society

There is a need to encourage society in general to recognise its positive role in the promotion of good health in children and their right to moral and material security. In addition to the provision of good material conditions of living, there is the responsibility of adults to examine critically the standards and example they set which influence children's decisions on matters of health such as smoking, sexual behaviour and drugs, and to re-establish as a high priority the prestige value of mothering and the stability of family life.

Appendix

Suggested Reading

General

May, E. D. 1980. *Community Paediatrics.* MTP Press Ltd.
Meadows, S. R. and Smithells, R. W. 1981. *Lecture Notes on Paediatrics.* Blackwell.
Meredith Davies, J. B. 1983. *Community Health and Social Services.* Hodder and Stoughton.
Meredith Davies, J. B. 1979. *Community Health, Preventive Medicine and Social Services.* Bailliere Tindall.
Mitchell, R. G. 1980. *Child Health in the Community.* Churchill Livingstone.

Chapter 1: Child, Family and Environment

Handbook of Contraceptive Practice. DHSS. 1979.
Neo-Natal Cold Injury. National Association for Maternal and Child Welfare. 1978.
Prevention and Health: Everybody's Business. HMSO. 1976.
Wedge, P. and Prosser, H. 1973. *Born to Fail.* Arrow.
Which Benefit? DHSS Leaflet FB/2. 1980.

Chapter 2: The Prevention of Communicable Disease

Control of Communicable Disease in School. DHSS. 1977.
Immunisation against Infectious Disease. DHSS. 1982.
Parry, W. H. 1979. *Communicable Diseases.* Hodder and Stoughton.

Chapter 3: Indices of Health

Emery, J. L. 1976. *Unexpected Death in Infancy.* Ch. 8 in *Recent Advances in Paediatrics, No. 5.* Ed. D. Hull. Churchill Livingstone.
Haemolytic Disease of the Newborn. DHSS. 1976.
Jackson, R. H., Ed. 1977. *Children, the Environment and Accidents.* Pitman.

Reducing the Risk: Safer Pregnancy and Childbirth. HMSO. 1977.
Wynn, M. and Wynn, A. 1976. *Prevention of Handicap of Perinatal Origin.* Foundation for Education and Research in Child-bearing.
Wynn, M. and Wynn, A. 1977. *The Prevention of Pre-term Birth.* Foundation for Education and Research in Child-bearing.

Chapters 4, 5, 6 and 7: Surveillance of Health

Bowlby, J. 1965. *Child Care and the Growth of Love.* Penguin.
Deafness in Early Childhood. DHSS. 1971.
Francis, D. E. M. 1975. *Diets for Sick Children.* Blackwell.
Illingworth, R. S. 1979. *The Normal Child.* Churchill Livingstone.
Illingworth, R. S. 1980. *Development of the Infant and Young Child, Normal and Abnormal.* Churchill Livingstone.
Illingworth, R. S. 1974. *The Child at School.* Blackwell.
McKinney, I. and Gordon, N. 1980. *Helping Clumsy Children.* Churchill Livingstone.
Screening for the Detection of Congenital Dislocation of the Hip. DHSS. 1969.
Sheridan, M. D. 1975. *The Developmental Progress of Infants and Young Children.* HMSO.
Valman, H. B. 1980. *The First Year of Life.* BMA Publications.
Winnicott, D. W. 1964. *The Child, the Family and the Outside World.* Pelican.

Chapter 8: Health Education

Breastfeeding. National Association for Maternal and Child Welfare. 1977.
Dallas, D. M. 1972. *Sex Education.* National Foundation for Educational Research.
Eating for Health. HMSO. 1978.
Lobo, E. de H. 1978. *Children of Immigrants in Britain.* Hodder and Stoughton.
My Body Project. The Health Education Council in association with the City of Sheffield Education Department. (To be published by Heinemann Educational Books in 1983).
Present Day Practice in Infant Feeding. HMSO Report on Health and Social Subjects Nos. 9 and 20. 1974 and 1980.

Chapter 9: Services for Children

1983 *Guide to Social Services.* Family Welfare Association. (This is an annual publication).

Illingworth, R. S. 1971. *Treatment of the Child at Home.* Blackwell.
Keywood, O. 1977. *Nursing in the Community.* Bailliere Tindall.
MacCarthy, D. 1979. *The Under-5s in Hospital.* National Association for the Welfare of Children in Hospital.
Owen, G. M., Ed. 1977. *Health Visiting.* Bailliere Tindall.
Penelope Hall's Social Services of England and Wales. Ed. J. Mays, A. Forder and O. Keidan. Routledge and Kegan Paul. 1975.
Slack, P. A. 1978. *School Nursing.* Bailliere Tindall.

Chapter 10: Children with Handicaps

Anderson, E. and Spain, B. 1977. *The Child with Spina Bifida.* Methuen.
Bowley, A. H. and Gardner, L. 1980. *The Handicapped Child.* Churchill Livingstone.
Cunningham, C. and Sloper, P. 1978. *Helping your Handicapped Baby.* Human Horizons Series. Souvenir Press.
Finnie, N. R. 1974. *Handling the Young Cerebral Palsied Child at Home.* Heinemann.
Furneaux, B. 1981. *The Special Child.* Pelican.
Hart, D. and Walters, J. 1979. *One of the Family.* The Disabilities Study Unit, Arundel.
Help for Handicapped People. DHSS Leaflet HB/1. 1981.
Hosking, G. 1981. *An Introduction to Paediatric Neurology.* Faber and Faber.
Human Genetics. DHSS. 1972.
Inheritance—a Guide to Genetic Counselling. National Association for Maternal and Child Welfare, 1980.
Jeffree, D. 1982. *Pathways to Independence.* Hodder and Stoughton.
Nolan, M. and Tucker, I. G. 1981. *The Hearing Impaired Child and the Family.* Human Horizons Series. Souvenir Press.
Russell, P. 1976. *Help Starts Here.* National Children's Bureau for the Voluntary Council for Handicapped Children.
Wing, L. 1971. *The Autistic Child.* Constable.

Chapter 11: Children in Special Circumstances

Bowskill, D. 1980. *Single Parents.* Futura.
Low Cost Day Provisions for the Under-Fives. Conference Papers. 1976. DHSS and DES. 1976.
Needs of the Under-5s in the Family. The Children's Committee. 1980.
Rutter, M. 1975. *Helping Troubled Children.* Pelican.
Rutter, M. 1981. *Maternal Deprivation Reassessed.* Pelican.
Wolff, S. 1981. *Children Under Stress.* Pelican.

Chapter 12: Non-Accidental Injury

Carter, J., Ed. 1974. *The Maltreated Child.* Priory Press.
O'Doherty, N. 1982. *The Battered Child.* Bailliere Tindall.

Chapter 13: Bereavement in the Family

Lonsdale, G., Elfer, P. and Ballard, R. 1979. *Children, Grief and Social Work.* Blackwell.
Rudolph, M. 1978. *Should the Children Know?* MTP Press.
Support and Counselling for Bereaved Parents. Foundations for the Study of Infant Deaths. 1978.
The Loss of Your Baby. Health Education Council. 1980.
What to do after a Death. DHSS Leaflet D/49.

Children and the Law

Hoggett, B. 1981. *Parents and Children.* Sweet and Maxwell.
Jackson, J., Book, M. and Hains, B., Ed. 1977 and supplement 1979. *Clarke Hall and Morrison's Law Relating to the Children and Young Persons.* Butterworth.
Jones, R. M., Ed. 1980. *Social Work Statutes.* Sweet and Maxwell.

Reports

Child Welfare Centres. (The Sheldon Report). HMSO. 1967.
* *Fit for the Future: The Report of the Committee on Child Health Services.* (The Court Report). HMSO. 1976.
Inequalities in Health. (The Black Report). HMSO. 1980.
Meeting Special Educational Needs. (Brief Guide). HMSO. 1980.
* *One-Parent Families.* (The Finer Report). HMSO. 1974.
Perinatal and Neonatal Mortality. (The Short Report). HMSO. 1980.
* *Special Educational Needs: Report of the Enquiry into the Education of Handicapped Children and Young People.* (The Warnock Report). HMSO. 1978.

* The National Children's Bureau Information Service produce excellent summaries in their 'Highlight' Series.

Index

Accidents 3, 63–6
Accidents and Emergency department
164
Acts
Adoption 217
Children 217
Clean Air 14
Family Planning 4
Midwives 51
Nurseries and Child Minders 213
Adolescence 118–119
Adoption 169, 216–221
Advice centres
benefits 211
housing 10
Aids
daily living 192
hearing 101, 184
mobility 184, 192
Air 13–14
Alcohol 53, 119, 148–9
Alpha-feto-protein 56, 202
Amniocentesis 56, 178, 199, 201
Anaemia
in pregnancy 55
iron-deficiency 94
sickle cell 95, 137
Anorexia nervosa 120
Ante-natal
care 2, 51, 55
health education 127, 178
screening 55–56
Asthma 113, 172–175
Audiometrician 69, 113, 182
Autism 103, 204

Behaviour disturbances 101, 107, 116,
119, 136, 155
Benefits
child 6
constant attendance allowance 190
death grant 234
family income supplement 6, 208

low income entitlement 6
maternity 208
mobility allowance 190
one-parent 6, 208
supplementary 6, 208
widowed mother 208
Bereavement
counselling 232–233, 235
practical help in 233
Blood examination 51–56, 94–95
Breast feeding 23, 57, 79, 129–131,
137

Carrier 20
Cataract, congenital 92
Census 47–48
Cerebral palsy 97, 98, 203
Chickenpox 31
Child care assistant 170, 196
Child health clinic 69, 153–154
Child minder 169, 193, 213–214
Circumcision 93
Clinical medical officer 156, 165, 182
Clumsy child 116
Coeliac disease 76
Cold injury 7
Colour blindness 113
Communicable disease 18 et seq.
contact tracing 23, 146
control of 21–30
notification of 22
Community health
council 168
services 61, 152–161
staff 23, 53, 62, 67, 156–160, 211
Community home 169, 194, 216
Congenital abnormality
deaths due to 60
notification of 49, 179
prevention of 61
screening for 56
Co-ordinated care 62, 67, 77, 87, 171–
175, 200, 212

Cot-death, *see* sudden infant death
Counselling
  adolescents 118-119, 189
  adoption 218
  bereavement 232-233
  genetic 77, 87, 178, 187, 202, 205
  handicap 186-189
Court orders
  adoption 217
  affiliation 209
  care 229
  maintenance 209
  place of safety 229
  supervision 230
Court Report 175-176
Cretinism, *see* hypothyroidism, congenital
Cystic fibrosis 76
Cytomegalic infection 45

Day care 169, 193, 212
Deafness 36, 100, 103, 113
Dehydration 33, 83
Dental
  caries 133
  health 133
  services 161
Department of Health 40, 47, 50
Depression, maternal 7, 208, 210
Diabetes 78, 113, 171-172, 173-175
Diet 71, 75, 79, 82, 128-135
  special 76, 77, 87, 155
  supplements 131
Dietitian 77, 124, 139, 160
Diphtheria 32
District Health Authority 27, 153
District medical officer 22, 48, 49, 123
District nursing service 159, 163, 174
Down's syndrome 56, 200
Drugs
  in pregnancy 128
  school children and 119, 149-151
Dysentery, Sonne 33

Eczema 94
Education
  department 6, 23, 67, 153, 169-170, 195, 200, 211
  social work service 170
  welfare officer 117, 170

Emotional influences 71, 79, 103, 112
Endocrine function 70-71, 79, 81, 88, 111
Enuresis 115, 155, 168
Environment
  affecting growth 74, 75, 79, 81-82
  family 1, 3
  intra-uterine 1-2
  post-natal 1, 3 et seq.
Environmental health department 8, 23
Epilepsy 113, 173-175
Ethnic minority groups 89-90, 137-139

Failure to thrive 74-75, 92
Family
  centres 169, 195
  environment 1, 3
  fund 191
  income 5-6
  life 138
  one-parent 207-210
  planning 4-5, 55, 129, 143, 189, 210, 225
  size 3-4
Feeding
  artificial 11, 131, 137
  breast 129-131, 137
  difficulties 75, 106
Fluoride
  and dental decay 134
  in water 13
Fontanelles 83
Food safety 11
Fostering 169, 194, 215-216
Full care 169, 194, 214-216, 229

Gastro-enteritis 32, 60, 78
General practitioner 62, 109, 117, 161-162, 174
  when to call 162-163
Gifted child 117, 121-122
Glue-ear 113
Grants
  death 234
  improvement 10, 192
  repair 10
Growth
  factors affecting 70

hormone deficiency 81, 111
measurement of 72–74
observation of 70, 111
variations of 74–82, 111
Guthrie test 86

Haemolytic streptococcal infection 11, 38
Haemophilia 1, 181, 205
Handicapped children
assessment of 181, 185
care facilities 193–195
education 195–198
financial help 190
housing help 191
identification 179–180
prevention 10, 177
register of 180
Handicap team 182–184
Head circumference 72, 73, 82
Health education
ante-natal 55, 127, 178
communicable disease 30
council 123
dental 133
department 123
ethnic minority groups 137–139
in early years 132–139
in schools 53, 139–151
obesity 112
officer 123
rickets 90
safety 64–65
Health services
community 61, 152–161
general practitioner 161–163
health education 123
hospital 164–167
maternity 55
psychiatric 165
school 154–156
Health
questionnaire 110
record 49, 62, 175
Health visitor 49, 62, 64–65, 157–159, 211
liaison 158, 182
special 174, 182
Hearing 101, 110, 113
Heart, congenital defect of 60, 92

Height 1, 4, 72, 73, 80–82, 111
Hepatitis, infective 34
Heredity 1
affecting growth 70, 79, 80, 103
Hernia, inguinal 92
Hip, congenital dislocation of 85–86
Home help 169, 193
Hospital
activity analysis 49
day unit 165
education in 166, 197
services 164, 173, 194
stay 165–166
visiting 166
Housing 7–10
department 8
standards 8
help in 10, 137, 191, 209
Hydrocephalus 82, 83
Hyperactivity 116
Hypernatraemia 12
Hypothyroidism, congenital 88

Illness
general 52, 71, 76, 81, 94
infectious 7, 60
Immunisation 26, 30
contra-indications to 27
programmes of 27, 28–29, 43
reactions to 27
Immunity 23–30
Immunoglobulin 23, 30, 34
Impetigo 41
Incubation period 20
Infant mortality 51–52

Lactose intolerance 77
Language
development 102
difficulties 137
Later childhood mortality 63–68
Lead
in environment 12, 14–15
poisoning 15, 95
Legal help 210
Leisure 192
Leukaemia 27, 67, 95
Lice, head 43
Local authority
care 215
departments 8, 10, 11, 12, 168–170

Locomotion
delay in 96
development of 96–97

Malignant diseases 67, 171
Manipulation
delay in 98
development of 98
Maternity
benefits 128
services 55
Measles 35
Medico-social history 69–70
Meningitis 35, 60
Mental retardation 36, 97, 98, 103, 202
Methaemoglobinaemia 13
Microcephalus 83
Midwife 55, 62, 130
community 159
Milk
breast 23
dried 11
free 6, 112, 128, 153, 155, 191
intolerance 78
safety of 11
MOEH 22, 23
Mongolism, *see* Down's syndrome
Multiple developmental delay 204
Mumps 36
Muscular dystrophy 204

Naevi 93
Nappy rash 93–94
Neo-natal care 56–57
New baby, preparation for 135
Nitrates 12
Non-accidental injury 222 et seq.
prevention of 222–226
procedure in 228–230
register 226
review committee 226
signs of 226–228
Notification
births 48
communicable disease 22, 49
congenital abnormality 49, 179
handicap 80
NSPCC 225–226, 229
Nursery
day 169, 193, 212, 213, 225

infection in 23
private 169
residential 194
surveillance in 69, 213
Nursery school 170, 195, 211, 214, 225
Nursing
equipment 163, 192
staff 67, 90, 182

Obesity 78–80, 112, 158
Occupational therapist 182
One-parent family 207–210
OPCS 47, 49
Orthoptist 69, 99, 182
Otitis media 35, 114, 162

Paediatrician 62, 67, 87, 174, 182
Parents 3, 62, 104–106, 124, 148–151,
163, 174, 183, 207, 210, 230
Percentile charts 73, 74, 80, 81, 83, 111
Perinatal mortality 53–57
Pertussis, *see* whooping cough
Phenylketonuria 1, 57, 86–87
Physical examination 88–89, 95, 112
Physiotherapist 160, 182
Plantar warts, *see* verrucae
Play 105–106, 138, 195, 225
Poliomyelitis 36–37
Post-perinatal mortality 58–63
Poverty 3, 211, 223
Preparation for
hospital 166
new baby 134
parenthood 146
school 135
Primary care team 161
Proper officer 22, 49
Psychiatrist, child 117, 165
Psychologist
clinical 165, 182
educational 69, 109, 117, 165, 174,
182
Psycho-social factors 75, 82, 111, 211,
223
Puberty 111

Rates
birth 48
death 48
illegitimate birth 48

infant mortality 48, 51–52
perinatal mortality 53
post-perinatal mortality 58
still-birth 48
Rebates 10, 208
Registration
    births 48
    deaths 48, 223
    still-birth 48, 223
Rehousing 10, 191
Relationships 57, 104–105, 133, 143
Respiratory infection 1, 7, 14, 60, 92
Rhesus incompatibility 55
Rickets 83, 89–90, 137
Rota viruses 45
Rubella 1, 37, 56, 100

Safety
    environmental 64–65, 137
    health education 65, 133, 135
Scabies 42
Scarlet fever 38
School
    attendance records 110, 121
    doctor 109, 111, 116, 174
    health service 136, 154–156, 174,
    196
    infection in 23
    meals service 77, 87, 135, 170
    nurse 75, 109, 113, 160, 174
    preparation for 135
    psychological service 117, 170
    refusal 121
Schoolgirl pregnancy 119–120
Schriver test 87
Scoliosis 114
Screening tests 55–56, 57, 85–88, 98–
    99, 101, 113–114
Sex education 141
Sexual problems 119
Sexually transmitted disease 55, 119,
    144–147
Short stature 80–82, 111
Sickle cell anaemia 95, 137
Skin 93–94
    infections 41–43
Sleep
    difficulties 107
    in school child 135
Smoking 1, 53, 119, 128, 147–148

Social
    development 103–105, 114
    disadvantage 210–211, 222
    services department 23, 67, 153,
    168–169
    worker 62, 67, 120, 165, 168, 174,
    182, 211, 230
Speech
    development 101–102
    indistinct 103
    therapist 69, 100, 109, 160, 182
Spina bifida 56, 97, 201
Squint 99
Stammer 103
Stimulation, lack of 97, 98, 103
Subdural haematoma 82, 228
Sudden infant death 60, 61–62
Suicide 121
Surveillance programmes 69, 96–97,
    109, 179
Swimming baths 13

Teachers 69, 90, 100, 116–117, 174,
    182, 195, 211
Teeth 95
Tetanus 38–39
Testes, undescended 93
Toilet training 107
Transmission of infection 18–19
Tuberculosis 11, 39

Understanding, development of 103–
    104

Verrucae 43
Visual
    handicap 100
    screening 99, 110, 113
Vitamin(s)
    deficiency 89–90
    free 6, 128, 155
Voluntary bodies 171, 212, 225

Warnock Report 196
Water 12–13
Weaning 131
Weight 72, 73, 112–113
Whooping cough 39–40
Working mothers 206